THE LEARNING IMPERATIVE

WHY MOST HEALTH SYSTEMS FAIL AND HOW YOURS WILL SUCCEED

NABIL ZARY

NeuroInk

The Learning Organization Imperative: Why Academic Health Systems Must Transform And How to Start

Published by NeuroInk Press

Book cover artwork by: Laila Bihmidine

1st Edition: December 2025

ISBN: 978-969-9893-54-4 (hardcover)

ISBN: 978-969-9893-55-1 (paperback)

ISBN: 978-969-9893-56-8 (ebook)

DISCLAIMER

This book offers general guidance on organizational transformation within academic health systems. It is not meant to serve as professional consulting advice tailored to your particular organization. The case studies and examples are composites drawn from various real situations, with details altered to ensure confidentiality. Any similarities to specific organizations or individuals are purely coincidental.

The author and publisher do not guarantee the accuracy, completeness, or suitability of this information. Organizational transformation presents complex challenges that vary by context. Readers are encouraged to perform their own assessments and, when necessary, consult professionals before making major organizational decisions.

The author and publisher explicitly disclaim any responsibility for liability, loss, or risk —personal or otherwise—that may arise directly or indirectly from using or applying any part of this book.

To the academic health system leaders who choose the hard path of genuine transformation over the easy path of transformation theater.

To the frontline clinicians and staff who deserve organizations worthy of their commitment.

And to the patients who trust us with their lives and deserve the best care our knowledge allows.

CONTENTS

FOREWORD

This book is based on a decade of experience working with academic health systems on transformation. I've observed dedicated leaders struggle not because of a lack of commitment or skill, but because they rely on ineffective methods. I wrote this to share lessons learned from both failures and successes—to help leaders understand why transformations often fail and what methods are truly effective. My goal is to offer honest guidance that encourages action, rather than just presenting inspiring theories. If this book enables even one academic health system to foster real learning, improve patient care, and create a positive work environment, it will have been worthwhile. Real change in academic medicine won't come from external consultants or plans alone, but from leaders like you making decisive choices and maintaining discipline over time.

This book shows you how. What you do with it is up to you.

Nabil Zary
December 2025

INTRODUCTION

WHAT YOU'LL LEARN, AND WHAT HAPPENS NEXT

WHY THIS BOOK EXISTS

Academic medicine is facing a crisis. It's not the urgent, headline-making kind that demands quick action. Instead, it's a subtle, gradually worsening problem that leads you to believe everything is under control until it suddenly isn't.

You are already aware of this. It shows up in your quality metrics, which remain stubbornly resistant to improvement despite numerous initiatives. It's evident in your workforce—physicians and nurses experiencing burnout at a rate faster than you can recruit new staff. It appears in your operating margins, which are so compressed that they threaten your ability to sustain the academic mission. And it's visible in the widening gap between what medical science knows and the actions your clinicians regularly take.

You've made efforts to tackle these issues through strategic plans, consultant engagements, lean transformations, high reliability initiatives, patient experience programs, and technology implementations. While each was initiated with optimism and investment, and some initial progress was achieved, they ultimately stalled or regressed as focus shifted to new priorities.

The issue isn't a lack of effort or dedication. Instead, it's that you're trying to implement twenty-first-century transformation with organizational models created for a different time. You're addressing systemic issues with isolated initiatives. What you truly need is to focus on building core capabilities.

This book is here because academic health systems require a different, effective, and sustainable approach. It offers more than just a framework to examine or an aspirational vision to aim for someday. Instead, it provides a practical roadmap for transformation that you can start implementing as early as tomorrow morning.

I wrote this after a decade working with academic health systems on transformation efforts. I've seen patterns repeat: the same mistakes, pitfalls, and preventable failures. At the same time, I've observed rare successes—organizations that genuinely develop lasting learning ability and achieve the outcomes others only discuss but seldom realize.

This book condenses those patterns into practical advice. It candidly explains why transformation often fails, clarifies what truly works, and is detailed enough for immediate use without further planning or preparation.

WHAT THIS BOOK IS (AND ISN'T)

This is not an exhaustive academic treatise on learning organizations. It isn't a 400-page textbook covering every theory and framework. Nor is it a collection of case studies that you read passively, only to return to your unchanged reality.

This is a call to action intended for busy leaders who must grasp the core message swiftly and proceed to execution without delay. It can be read in two to three hours, leaving you clear on the next steps, their importance, and how to initiate them.

This book outlines five specific promises to you...

First, it tells the truth. This isn't the sanitized, politically correct version found in most healthcare management books. It reveals the real reasons behind why your past transformation efforts failed, what is truly wrong in your organization, and why fixing it will be more difficult than you might hope. If you're looking for reassurance that you're already doing well and only need minor adjustments, you can close this book now. But if you're prepared for honest, even uncomfortable, insights, continue reading.

Second, it's immediately actionable. Each chapter concludes with clear next steps you can take, such as "schedule this meeting by this date with these people to make this decision," rather than vague suggestions like "consider developing a strategy." By the end of Chapter 4, you'll have a detailed 90-day implementation plan. After finishing the book, you'll know your top three actions for tomorrow morning.

Third, it's grounded in reality. The examples and case studies are drawn from real academic health systems—anonymized when needed but always authentic. The timelines reflect real-world scenarios, not idealized goals. The resource needs are transparently communicated. Challenges are acknowledged without downplaying them. If a process requires 18 months, I will tell you it takes 18 months and explain why shortcuts tend to fail.

Fourth, it focuses on governance. This is the core argument of the book and a significant shift from standard transformation literature. While most books focus on culture, leadership, or methodology, this book contends that without clear governance—defined as explicit authority structures and decision rights—nothing else is effective. Governance is not just one component; it serves as the fundamental basis that either facilitates or hinders all other efforts. You'll dedicate an entire chapter to exploring governance models and determining the appropriate governance approach for your organization.

Fifth, it emphasizes capability over initiatives. This book doesn't provide a new improvement program to start. Instead, it teaches you how to develop organizational capability for ongoing learning that remains effective regardless of initiatives. The focus isn't on deploying PDSA, Lean, or Six Sigma specifically, but on cultivating a systematic ability to recognize problems, test solutions, evaluate results, and share effective practices—using whatever methods suit your situation.

> THE UNCOMFORTABLE TRUTH
>
> *Most people who buy books about organizational transformation never implement anything from them. The book becomes a substitute for action—proof that you're "taking transformation seriously" without the risk of actually changing anything. This book is valuable only if you do something with it. Otherwise, it's expensive reassurance.*

WHO SHOULD READ THIS BOOK

This book primarily targets senior leaders in academic health systems—such as CEOs, CMOs, CNOs, deans, hospital presidents, and board members—who have the authority to make strategic decisions about organizational change. If you can allocate resources, create governance frameworks, and define strategic directions, then this book is relevant for you.

But it also benefits anyone leading transformation efforts, even without formal authority. Quality improvement directors will gain practical advice on developing QI skills beyond just training. Department chairs will learn how to involve their teams in systematic improvements. Project directors and transformation officers will receive clear roadmaps for execution. Even frontline clinicians and staff will benefit from insights into why transformations often fail and what true success entails.

No prior expertise in learning organizations, quality improvement, or organizational development is required. The book explains concepts clearly without assuming specialized knowledge. You don't need to have read Peter Senge or studied the literature on learning health systems. It offers essential context while maintaining a focus on practical application.

What you truly need is the authority to make decisions or influence others, along with the willingness to face uncomfortable truths about your organization. If you can effect change—or can influence those who do—and are prepared to hear honest evaluations even when they challenge your assumptions, this book will be valuable to you.

WHAT YOU'LL LEARN

The book presents a logical sequence, starting with understanding the problem and moving to implementing the solution.

Chapter 1: The Crisis in Academic Medicine highlights four interconnected crises: persistent quality and safety gaps despite medical advances, workforce burnout and departure caused by organizational issues, financial instability jeopardizing the academic mission, and the seventeen-year delay in translating evidence into practice. These are not separate problems, but failures of organizational capability that are linked.

Chapter 2: Why Transformation Efforts Fail identifies five common mistakes made in nearly every transformation and highlights a fundamental structural flaw that causes all of them. You will see familiar patterns from your own unsuccessful projects. More crucially, you'll grasp the core issue—the governance gap—that explains why even well-funded and well-intentioned efforts often fall short.

Chapter 3: The Governance Decision outlines three effective governance models for developing a learning organization: centralized (emphasizing control and consistency), federated (focusing on speed and local adaptation), and hub-and-spoke (striking a balance between the two). You will explore decision criteria to select the appropriate model for your context, understand each model's benefits and costs, and learn how to implement your chosen model with real authority instead of just governance theater.

Chapter 4: The First 90 Days offers weekly guidance for your initial implementation phase. You'll learn to ensure governance is genuine, conduct honest readiness assessments, develop a vision through dialogue rather than top-down orders, and create strategic quick wins that showcase value and build momentum. By the end of this chapter, you'll have a clear action plan for your first three months.

Chapter 5: The Three Essential Capabilities outline the fundamental infrastructure you need to establish: psychological safety that allows people to learn from failures without fear, mentoring for quality improvement that develops skills through apprenticeship, and data-driven learning cycles that connect practice, insight, and action. You will see why all three are essential and how they are interconnected.

Chapter 6: Common Pitfalls reveals how organizations can undermine successful transformations. You'll learn to identify and steer clear of six common mistakes: declaring victory prematurely, tolerating toxic high performers, letting governance weaken, underinvesting in capability renewal, scaling prematurely, and engaging in measurement theater that focuses on metrics rather than outcomes.

Conclusion: Your Transformation Starts Now distills everything into straightforward choices and quick steps. You'll walk away with a precise plan for what to do tomorrow morning and in the coming months.

HOW TO USE THIS BOOK

If you have two to three hours, read from start to finish without skipping. The chapters are logically connected, and the foundation chapters set the necessary context for understanding the more practical implementation sections.

If you're short on time or need to persuade others before diving in fully, begin with Chapter 1 (the crisis) and Chapter 2 (why you're failing). These two chapters alone will change how you view transformation challenges. If they resonate with you, proceed to the implementation chapters.

If you're experiencing difficulties during a transformation, refer straight to Chapter 6 (common pitfalls). You will likely identify the mistakes you're making and be able to adjust your approach promptly.

If you're a board member or executive seeking to grasp the strategic reasoning without delving into implementation specifics, review Chapter 1 (the crisis), Chapter 2 (why transformation fails), and Chapter 3 (governance decision). These chapters lay out the strategic case and outline the key decision you need to make.

As you go through this, keep a pen handy. Highlight parts that stand out to you. Jot down questions that come up. Identify actions for your organization. This isn't a book for passive reading and then setting aside. It's a practical document to mark up, review often, and share with your leadership team.

After completing the book, visit LearningOrgPlaybook.com for additional resources, including assessment tools, implementation templates, and case studies. The book offers your roadmap, while the website supplies supportive tools for the process.

WHAT HAPPENS AFTER YOU FINISH

By the end of this book, you'll have a clear understanding of three key points.

First, you'll understand why you've been failing. Not due to a lack of commitment, resources, or talent. Instead, you've been repeating predictable structural errors that ensure failure despite your efforts. Recognizing this is freeing—it shows that success is achievable when you tackle the root causes rather than just the symptoms.

Second, you'll know exactly what to do. No vague principles to consider—just specific decisions, actions, capabilities, and pitfalls. You will receive a 90-day roadmap and guidance for the next 18 to 36 months of sustained effort required for true transformation.

Third, you'll face a choice. Continue engaging in transformation theater that generates activity but no real results. Accept reduced ambitions and step back from the academic mission. Alternatively, dedicate yourself to genuinely developing a learning organization over the years required to achieve success. The book clarifies the choice but leaves the decision to you.

Your next step will vary based on your decision.

If you opt for genuine transformation, your initial three steps are: schedule the governance conversation within two weeks, perform an honest readiness assessment within 30 days, and identify strategic quick wins within 60 days. Completing these three tasks marks the start.

If you opt to maintain the status quo or lower your ambitions, be transparent about it. Avoid starting initiatives you cannot sustain, and refrain from exhausting your workforce with what amounts to transformational theatrics. Take responsibility for your choice.

The change that academic medicine requires won't come from another initiative, consultant, or strategic plan. Instead, it will occur as organizations like yours make focused decisions, develop core capabilities, and stay committed over many years.

This book shows you how. What you do with it is up to you.

BEFORE YOU BEGIN

This book makes demands of its readers. Before you invest two to three hours, consider whether you're prepared to meet them.

1. Why are you reading this book? Be specific. If your answer involves words like "explore," "consider," or "learn about," you may be using reading as a substitute for action. Transformation books are often purchased by people who want to feel like they're doing something without actually doing anything.

2. Who assigned this to you, or did you choose it yourself? If someone else asked you to read it, do they have the authority to act on its recommendations? If you chose it yourself, do you have that authority—or are you hoping to convince someone who does?

3. Think of the last organizational change initiative you were part of. Did it succeed? If not, do you know why it failed? If you can't answer that question honestly, this book will give you another initiative to fail at.

4. What are you prepared to give up? Transformation requires stopping some things to start others. If you're planning to add learning and organizational development on top of everything you're already doing, you're setting yourself up to fail.

5. Are you reading this book hoping it will confirm decisions you've already made, or are you genuinely open to discovering you've been approaching transformation wrong?

If these questions made you uncomfortable, good. That discomfort is the beginning of honest self-assessment.

Now let's begin.

PART I

THE PROBLEM

1

THE CRISIS IN ACADEMIC MEDICINE

THE FOUR CONVERGING CRISES YOU'RE FACING AND WHY THEY'RE GETTING WORSE

THE CALL

At 11:47 PM, my phone rang, and it was the CEO of a major academic medical center—someone I'd known for years—who sounded exhausted.

She spoke softly, "This is our third preventable death this month." The issue is the same—central line infections that should never occur. Despite having protocols, training, and dashboards monitoring compliance, we find ourselves again having to inform another family that their loved one died from a preventable cause.

She paused. "I don't understand. We're meant to be an elite academic medical center, with brilliant physicians and world-class researchers, ranked nationally. How can we still be causing harm through basic infection control failures?"

I have explored this topic in various discussions with leaders at academic health systems on three different continents. While each institution faces unique issues, they all share the same fundamental confusion: how can they be both excellent and failing simultaneously?

The reality is more unsettling than many leaders admit. Academic medicine is confronting multiple crises that existing organizational structures cannot resolve. We attempt to tackle 21st-century issues using governance, culture, and operational models rooted in a vastly different past. Each year we postpone essential reforms, resulting in increased patient suffering, clinician burnout, and health systems nearing financial collapse.

This isn't an exaggeration. It's the reality you're experiencing, even if you haven't identified it yet.

I'll begin by illustrating the four crises currently impacting academic health systems. Then, I'll explain why previous efforts haven't succeeded—and what approaches will actually work.

CRISIS ONE: THE QUALITY AND SAFETY GAP

Medical knowledge has progressed more in the last twenty years than in the previous two centuries. We can now cure cancers that once seemed deadly just a generation ago. Additionally, we can replace failing organs and target therapies with precision at the molecular level. This scientific progress is truly remarkable.

Preventable medical errors continue to be a significant cause of death in the U.S. Estimates suggest that 200,000 to 400,000 lives are lost each year due to these errors—more than deaths from motor accidents, breast cancer, and AIDS combined. Despite knowing how to prevent many hospital-acquired infections, they still cause tens of thousands of deaths. Medication errors that should be avoidable still cause harm to hundreds of thousands of patients. Diagnostic errors, such as missed or delayed diagnoses, impact millions.

This isn't about a lack of medical knowledge. We understand what methods are effective. Evidence-based guidelines are available for nearly every common condition. We know how to prevent central line infections, reduce surgical complications, manage sepsis, and prevent medication errors. The disconnect isn't between our knowledge and scientific possibilities. Instead, the gap lies between what we know and what we reliably practice.

Academic health systems need to bridge this gap. With your

research expertise, you can identify best practices. Your educational missions are crucial for training future professionals. Additionally, your advanced data systems enable performance tracking. These systems should serve as laboratories of excellence, where innovation is quickly tested, proven practices are systematically adopted, and ongoing learning continuously enhances improvement.

Most academic health systems tend to follow a troubling pattern: isolated centers of excellence surrounded by widespread mediocrity. One department may deliver outstanding results while an adjacent one struggles with fundamental quality issues. Successful innovations in pilot projects rarely expand beyond their initial setting. Improvement efforts often start with enthusiasm, demonstrate early success, but then gradually diminish as focus shifts to other priorities.

Persistent and unwarranted variation exists in healthcare. Patients treated for the same condition within the same system often face vastly different outcomes depending on factors such as the physician they see, the unit of admission, or the day they arrive. This disparity isn't due to differences in patient severity or complexity. However, it stems from which team is providing care and whether that team has adopted current best practices or is still using outdated methods learned twenty years ago.

I have observed this pattern repeatedly in various institutions. A top cardiology team develops a groundbreaking heart failure protocol that lowers readmissions by 30%. Yet, three years later, this protocol remains confined to cardiology. The broader medicine team, which handles many more heart failure cases, has not adopted it. When I inquire about the reasons, the answers are consistently troubling: "We heard about it, but our patients are different," "We're planning to explore it next year," and "We tried something similar before, and it didn't work."

Translation: Knowledge remains confined within departmental silos, preventing innovation from spreading. As a result, patients continue to suffer from issues we've already addressed—just not within their specific unit.

This gap in quality and safety isn't merely a clinical issue; it's a moral failing. Each preventable death, avoidable complication, and delayed diagnosis signifies a patient who relied on us to provide the best evidence-based care but received less. The divide between our knowledge and action is reflected in lives lost and extended suffering.

THE UNCOMFORTABLE TRUTH

You already know which physicians in your organization are causing preventable harm. You also know why they're still practicing without meaningful intervention. The question isn't whether this is happening—it's whether you're willing to do something about it.

CRISIS TWO: WORKFORCE BURNOUT AND EXODUS

Academic medicine is losing talent rapidly. Around 50% of physicians experience burnout, reporting emotional exhaustion, depersonalization, and a diminished sense of achievement. Some healthcare systems see nursing turnover rates surpassing 20% each year. Early-career faculty are leaving academic roles for private practice or industry at concerning levels. Medical students are increasingly shying away from primary care, not because of a lack of interest, but because they observe residents and faculty overwhelmed by administrative tasks, moral distress, and constant pressure to produce.

The human toll is severe. Talented clinicians, initially motivated to help people, now find themselves overwhelmed by excessive documentation, irrelevant quality metrics, and administrative duties that take valuable time away from patients. This leads to moral injury—the psychological damage caused by delivering care that contradicts their core values and training. They understand what patients require but are unable to meet those needs due to the limitations of the existing system.

This isn't just about individual resilience or self-care; it's about how organizational dysfunction creates unsustainable working conditions. For example, when electronic health records focus on billing, they divert more physician attention from patient conversations, indicating an organizational failure. Similarly, when nurses spend more time documenting rather than providing direct care, it reflects a systemic issue. Additionally, residents working hundred-hour weeks despite knowing that fatigue endangers both patients and clinicians signifies a leadership failure.

The financial burden is also significant. Replacing one physician can cost between $500,000 and $1 million, including recruitment, onboarding, lost productivity, and relationship disruptions. For large health systems, annual nursing turnover amounts to tens of millions of dollars. However, the more profound cost is the loss of expertise and institutional knowledge. When experienced clinicians depart, they carry with them years of accumulated wisdom about effective practices in your specific environment, workflow efficiencies, and informal workarounds that help deliver patient care despite systemic barriers.

Organizations that tackle burnout through individual solutions—such as resilience training, meditation apps, or wellness committees—fail to address the root issue. Burnout isn't due to a lack of mindfulness; it stems from organizational factors that prevent meaningful work. You can't resolve systemic problems solely with wellness programs.

The workforce crisis is projected to worsen. Demographic trends will continue to cause shortages of physicians in primary care, psychiatry, and various specialties. Nursing shortages will increase as more experienced nurses retire before new graduates can replace them. Competition for talent will intensify, and health systems that struggle to retain staff will face severe staffing shortages.

Academic health systems are well-positioned to tackle this challenge. They manage medical education and can modify training programs to better equip clinicians for modern practice. Their research strengths allow them to discover and assess effective solutions. Furthermore, their missions are clearly centered on ongoing learning and development.

Instead, you exacerbate the problem by overloading staff with numerous initiatives. You introduce new documentation requirements faster than you remove outdated ones. Although you commend innovation, you punish the workflow disruptions caused by experimentation. You mention psychological safety, but let toxic behaviors from high-revenue clinicians continue.

The outcome: top talent exits, leaving remaining staff feeling cynical. This leads to a cycle in which you question why change initiatives fail, even when your team is too exhausted and demoralized to participate.

THE UNCOMFORTABLE TRUTH

Your best nurses don't leave for better pay. They leave because they can't do their jobs properly, and leadership keeps adding requirements without removing anything. Every time someone tells you "we just need to work smarter," they're blaming frontline staff for systemic failures.

CRISIS THREE: FINANCIAL UNSUSTAINABILITY

Operating margins at academic medical centers have been narrowing for years, with many systems functioning on very slim margins—only 1-3% during good years. The COVID-19 pandemic severely impacted even well-managed institutions, and some have yet to recover financially. The transition to value-based payment models eliminates the ability to offset operational inefficiencies through increased volume. Additionally, reimbursement from commercial payers is not keeping pace with rising costs, while government payment rates stay flat or decline.

Meanwhile, costs keep rising. Labor expenses rise due to workforce shortages, driving higher wages and costly agency staffing. Technology expenditures increase, with new electronic health record systems costing between $100 million to $500 million, excluding ongoing maintenance and improvements. Pharmaceutical expenses continue to rise. Infrastructure demands continuous investment. Community benefit and safety net responsibilities require resources regardless of reimbursement.

Academic health systems encounter specific financial challenges. They subsidize education, with teaching hospitals incurring significant expenses for resident and student training that are not entirely reimbursed. They also perform research, typically funded by grants that do not cover all costs. Additionally, they operate specialized, often unprofitable services such as burn units, trauma centers, and complex pediatric care that serve their mission. Furthermore, they offer charity care to uninsured and underinsured patients at higher levels than most community hospitals.

These mission-driven activities are vital, but they are financially unsustainable with current models. Essentially, you are subsidizing national benefits—such as training the future workforce, advancing medical knowledge, and offering safety net care—using operating margins from clinical revenue. When those margins disappear, the entire system fails.

The usual strategy has been to lower costs through broad cuts, hiring freezes, and efficiency efforts focused on minor improvements. However, these methods tend to yield diminishing returns and can negatively affect quality and staff morale. Achieving financial sustainability without sacrificing academic excellence requires more than just cutbacks.

What you need is essential waste reduction and value generation through operational change. Most health systems squander 30-50% of resources on activities that fail to enhance patient outcomes—such as duplicated tasks, preventable complications, unnecessary readmissions, inefficient workflows, and coordination issues. To cut this waste and boost quality, organizations must develop the ability for ongoing improvement. This skill doesn't come simply from hiring consultants or launching new initiatives; it involves becoming a learning organization.

Financial pressures are set to grow, with payment models increasingly prioritizing value over volume. Competition will intensify as new players—such as tech firms, retail clinics, and specialized providers—gain profitable service lines. Academic health systems that fail to overhaul their operating models risk declining margins, diminished mission capacity, and potentially existential threats.

CRISIS FOUR: THE EVIDENCE-TO-PRACTICE CHASM

Medical knowledge doubles roughly every seventy-three days, with thousands of research studies published each month. Clinical practice guidelines are constantly updated, and breakthrough therapies appear regularly. The speed of scientific progress has never been quicker.

On average, it takes seventeen years for research discoveries to become standard in clinical practice. Seventeen years from confirming "this works" to regularly applying it. This isn't just a delay—it's a wide gap. Patients are dying from treatable conditions because medical practice remains outdated, often years behind the latest medical knowledge.

Academic health systems must excel at quickly translating evidence into practice. You produce a significant portion of the research, and your faculty are thought leaders. Your team also possesses expertise in implementation science. The goal should be to narrow the evidence-to-practice gap, rather than highlight it.

Instead, you encounter the same translation challenges as others. Researchers produce findings that rarely reach clinicians. Clinicians are too busy to review the literature that could improve their practice. Electronic health records, created mainly for documentation, fail to deliver evidence effectively at the point of care. Protocols and guidelines are increasing rapidly, making it hard to keep up. Evidence-based practices often compete with long-standing habits, traditions, and the way things have always been done.

Patients at academic medical centers often receive care based on their physician's training and exposure. This care may not always align with current evidence, as it depends on the practices their doctors learned decades ago, along with any continuing education and guidelines they've encountered.

This issue isn't about whether individual physicians are competent. Even the most talented and dedicated clinicians cannot keep up with the rapidly growing medical knowledge while managing patient care, teaching, and research. The core problem is systemic. We require organizational systems that can consistently identify relevant evidence, critically assess it, quickly apply practice changes, and integrate new knowledge into workflows—ideally while the evidence is still recent, not after seventeen years.

Learning organizations develop this ability by systematically reviewing evidence, testing promising practices, measuring outcomes, and disseminating effective methods. They reduce the time from evidence to practice from 17 years to just 17 weeks, or even 17 days. This isn't due to individual clinicians working harder, but rather to organizational systems that translate evidence systematically rather than relying on chance.

THE UNCOMFORTABLE TRUTH

Your organization publishes research that you don't implement in your own clinical practice. Patients at your academic medical center receive care based on outdated evidence while your researchers publish the updated evidence that other organizations might eventually use. This is indefensible, and everyone knows it.

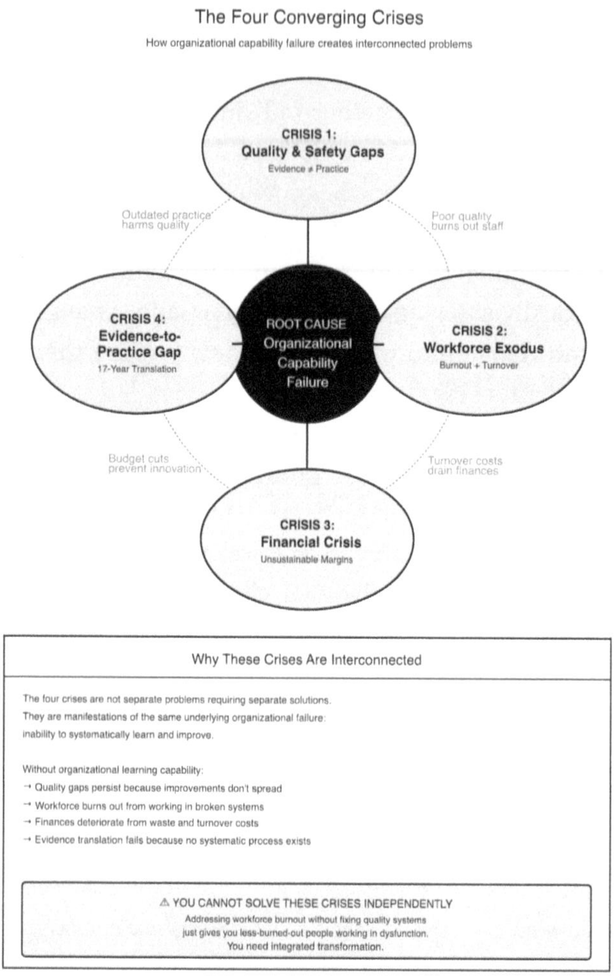

THE CONVERGENCE

Four crises: quality gaps, workforce exodus, financial instability, and failures in evidence translation. Each one requires urgent action; collectively, they pose an existential threat.

What makes this moment especially risky is that these crises are interconnected and reinforce each other. Poor quality leads to preventable complications, raising costs and adding stress to the workforce. Burnout among staff reduces quality and increases turnover costs. Financial stress prompts cost-cutting measures that worsen staff burnout and decrease investments in quality improvement. Failure to translate evidence keeps quality gaps unresolved and results in resource waste on ineffective practices.

You cannot tackle these crises in isolation. Fixing workforce burnout without addressing quality issues leaves staff less burned out but still delivering inconsistent care. Focusing solely on quality improvement without addressing workforce conditions leads to quicker burnout. Cutting costs with conventional efficiency methods often worsens both quality and staff experience. Pushing evidence into practice faster without enhancing learning capacity can cause initiative fatigue.

You require a comprehensive transformation that tackles all four crises at once through fundamental organizational change. This is not just another initiative, consultant engagement, or strategic plan with an inspiring vision but lacking effective implementation.

You must transform into a learning organization—one that consistently learns from each patient encounter, quickly applies evidence in practice, steadily enhances quality and efficiency, and fosters an environment where talented individuals are motivated to work.

This isn't just an optional upgrade; it's an essential requirement for existence.

THE STAKES

If you succeed in developing a learning organization, the following become achievable: quality gaps gradually narrow and eventually disappear as innovations are systematically spread rather than remaining isolated. Preventable deaths and complications decrease as evidence-based practices become the norm rather than the exception. Workforce engagement increases as employees find their work meaningful rather than burdensome, recognize that improvement initiatives succeed rather than fail, and work within psychologically safe environments rather than toxic cultures.

Financial performance improves as waste reduction generates margins that can be reinvested into the mission. Evidence quickly moves from discovery to application, establishing you as a genuine leader in medical advancement rather than a follower. The academic mission thrives through the integration of research, education, and clinical care around continuous learning, rather than functioning as separate entities.

If you fail to adapt—by sticking to usual practices, launching initiatives that don't last, trying to transform without establishing necessary foundations, or maintaining governance structures that hinder change—the consequences are clear: persistent and growing quality gaps as other organizations advance, ongoing preventable harm, an accelerated workforce exodus leading to staffing crises, shrinking financial margins making mission-driven activities unaffordable, and widening gaps between evidence and practice resulting in increasingly outdated care.

Ultimately, you must decide between abandoning the academic mission to ensure financial survival or upholding it at the risk of insolvency. Some institutions will prioritize survival and stop functioning as true academic health systems. Conversely, others will stay committed to their mission but confront financial crises.

A third option exists: transforming into a true learning organization that excels clinically, financially, and academically, as learning capability provides a competitive edge.

However, that approach involves examining why your earlier transformation efforts failed. This is the focus of the next chapter.

BEFORE YOU CONTINUE

These questions have no comfortable answers. If you can answer them easily, you're probably not being honest.

1. How many preventable deaths occurred in your organization last year? If you don't know the number immediately, what does that tell you about what your organization actually pays attention to?

2. When was the last time you personally heard a frontline nurse describe what's actually broken in your organization? Not in a survey. Not filtered through management. When did you last sit with a nurse and ask, "What makes your job harder than it should be?" And when was the last time you acted on what you heard?

3. If your most talented physician announced tomorrow that they were leaving for a competitor, would they cite organizational dysfunction as a reason? Would you believe them if they said no?

4. You've probably launched multiple improvement initiatives in the past five years. Name one that is still active and producing measurable results. If you can't name one, what does that pattern tell you?

5. Be honest: Have you already decided this transformation will be "different," or are you reading this book hoping it will confirm what you already want to do? The difference matters more than you think.

2

WHY TRANSFORMATION EFFORTS FAIL

THE FIVE PREDICTABLE MISTAKES AND THE ONE ROOT CAUSE THAT MAKES THEM ALL INEVITABLE

THE PATTERN

Three months ago, the CEO of a renowned academic medical center called me.

We've exhausted all options, she admitted, frustration clear in her voice. "Lean consultants. Six Sigma training. We've invested millions and trained hundreds of employees. Yet, after eighteen months, nothing has truly improved. What are we missing?"

I've had this very same conversation numerous times with leaders at academic health systems globally. Different institutions, sizes, and markets—yet the story remains the same.

The answer is always the same: they are not doing anything "wrong" in the usual sense. They make five common mistakes that nearly every transformation attempt involves—and overlook the one structural adjustment that makes all the difference.

Over the past decade, I have collaborated extensively with academic health systems undergoing transformation—ranging from 300-bed community teaching hospitals to large tertiary centers with billion-dollar budgets. I have seen visionary CEOs initiate bold projects, witnessed millions spent on consultants, training, and infrastructure, and observed the early excitement, pilot successes, and confident board presentations.

And repeatedly, I've seen these transformations not succeed.

It's not a matter of "partially succeeding" or "achieving some objectives." The organization fails. After three years, the same issues still exist. The silos are still in place, and the organization has shifted its focus to the next initiative.

The only ones who succeeded—fewer than you might think—did something genuinely different. And it wasn't what you'd typically expect.

These are the five main pitfalls. If you're truthful, you'll see at least three in your own organization.

KILLER #1: TOOL OBSESSION MEETS INITIATIVE PROLIFERATION

The most common pattern I observe begins with a prestigious academic medical center choosing to "implement Lean." They engage consultants in a multimillion-dollar project. Over the past two years, they have trained hundreds of staff in value stream mapping, 5S, and Kanban boards. They hold rapid-improvement events with significant publicity. Staff become certified, and leaders gain dashboards. Eventually, the consultants depart.

After three years, I come back to assess the impact. The tools are missing, the kanban boards are gone, the 5S protocols have been abandoned, and the metrics have returned to their original state. When I inquire with frontline staff about Lean, they dismiss it with eye rolls. "Oh, that was two initiatives ago. Now we're working on High Reliability."

What caused these transformations to fail? They focused on implementing tools but neglected to change the culture. They mapped value streams without tackling underlying power dynamics. They conducted improvement events without fostering psychological safety. They initiated new projects without phasing out the old ones.

The core mistake was assuming that teaching correct methods and launching numerous initiatives would automatically change behavior. However, essential questions were overlooked: Do people feel comfortable voicing concerns about processes created by senior physicians? Are department chairs encouraged to collaborate or compete? Does your promotion system prioritize systems improvement over individual publications? Most importantly, what are you prepared to give up to make space for new initiatives?

I've seen the effects of this obsession firsthand. During a site visit, a system CEO walked me through his organization's "strategic priorities." He began listing: Lean transformation, patient experience initiative, high-reliability organization efforts, physician wellness programs, nurse retention initiatives, population health expansion, EHR optimization, value-based care preparation, community health needs assessment, and research infrastructure development. He finally paused, visibly embarrassed. "I can't actually remember them all without checking my email."

During my interview with frontline staff at that institution, a nurse manager summed it up nicely: "Every six months, there's a new thing—new acronym, new training, new consultants. We smile, nod, and wait for it to pass because it always does."

How can you tell if you're making this mistake? Pay attention to how people discuss improvement efforts. If they say "We're doing Lean this year"—treating it as a project with a fixed deadline rather than a continuous operating philosophy—you might have an issue. If you can't easily list all your active strategic initiatives without looking at documentation, you likely have too many. If your board praises training completion rates more than actual patient outcomes, you're focusing on activity rather than impact. And if frontline staff greet new programs with exhausted cynicism, it shows they've learned that initiatives are just temporary distractions from real work.

Being busy doesn't necessarily mean you're making progress; simply staying busy isn't the same as achieving meaningful change.

THE UNCOMFORTABLE TRUTH

You don't have an initiative problem; you have a stopping problem. Your organization knows how to start new things but not how to stop old things. Every new initiative adds burden without removing burden. Eventually, "transformation" becomes just another thing people wait out.

KILLER #2: SILOED EXCELLENCE

Academic health systems tend to be organizationally fragmented. Department chairs focus on developing their own departments, which are evaluated based on research funding, clinical income, and reputation. They vie for resources, space, and talent. Medical, nursing, and allied health schools each have their own deans, budgets, and strategic goals. Additionally, hospitals and faculty practices frequently operate under separate governance frameworks and financial motives.

This design fosters excellence within each silo. The Department of Medicine specializes in hospital medicine. Surgery leads in surgical outcomes. The School of Nursing excels in nurse education. Each area accomplishes remarkable achievements.

However, silos hinder organizational learning.

I observed this pattern at a prominent academic medical center on the East Coast. The Department of Medicine implemented an innovative strategy to decrease hospital-acquired infections—remarkably, they reduced their HAI rates by 40% within six months. However, during my visit six months afterward, I toured the surgical units and found the same infection issues and persistent rates that had troubled them for years.

I asked the surgical leadership team, "Did you hear about Medicine's breakthrough?"

They had. "Yeah, we heard something about it," one surgeon said. "But surgery is different. What works in Medicine won't work here."

The intervention focused on universal infection-control principles, including hand hygiene, environmental cleaning, and catheter-care bundles. These evidence-based practices are applicable in all clinical settings and are not specific to Medicine. However, strong tribal identity—the belief that "our department is fundamentally different"—hindered the transfer of this knowledge.

Meanwhile, I found that five distinct departments were each tackling readmission reduction separately. There were five teams, five approaches, five data systems, and no collaboration or shared learning. The same problem was being addressed five times instead of just once.

This is the actual cost of siloed excellence. Innovation is confined to individual departments rather than spreading across the organization. Resources are duplicated among disconnected teams. System-wide issues, such as patient flow across different units, remain unresolved because no single entity owns the entire system—only their own segment. While each part may achieve excellence, the overall system results in mediocrity.

How can you tell if this is hindering your transformation? Listen for the phrase "That's interesting, but our department is different" whenever someone proposes adopting another unit's innovation. Observe whether different departments use different EHR templates to document the same clinical workflows. Notice whether your improvement meetings highlight individual department successes instead of system-wide changes. See if cross-department collaboration relies on heroic personal efforts rather than standard procedures. Finally, track whether successful pilot projects spread beyond their initial unit promptly or remain isolated victories that never expand.

When knowledge remains confined within departmental boundaries, it indicates you haven't established a true learning organization. Instead, you've created a set of isolated learning units that happen to share a brand name.

THE UNCOMFORTABLE TRUTH

When a department says "our patients are different" to avoid adopting another department's successful innovation, they're usually not protecting patients—they're protecting autonomy. The phrase "our patients are different" has become the socially acceptable way to say "we don't want to change."

KILLER #3: THE VOLUNTARY PARTICIPATION TRAP

This is a typical conversation I've had at almost every academic health system I've worked with. I meet with the Chief Quality Officer or the person responsible for improvement efforts to review their latest transformation initiative.

I ask, "How do you determine which departments take part?"

They explain, "We invite all departments to join; those interested can opt in."

And what about those who don't choose to opt in?

A pause. "We continually encourage them and share success stories from participating departments, hoping they'll recognize the value and join eventually."

This is the voluntary participation trap, and it's deadly. When transformation is framed as voluntary, it attracts only those willing to change, leaving the most in need of change out. High-performing departments tend to join because ongoing improvement fits their existing culture. In contrast, struggling departments often opt out because they feel overwhelmed, resistant, or convinced their issues are unique.

I observed this process at a West Coast academic medical center as it implemented a system-wide sepsis protocol. The protocol was evidence-based, well-structured, and had demonstrated success in early-adopting departments. After six months, seven departments had adopted it, while five had not. When asked about the holdouts, the responses were telling: "Our patient population is different," "We're not sure the evidence applies to our specialty," and "We're too busy with other priorities right now."

The tragic irony is that three of the five departments not participating had the highest sepsis mortality rates in the system. The departments most in need of the protocol were the ones refusing to adopt it. Meanwhile, the transformation team focused its efforts on high-performing departments that were likely to improve regardless.

Voluntary participation has a harmful side effect: it makes it impossible to determine if your intervention is effective. When only motivated departments join, any improvements might be due to their inherent culture of excellence rather than the intervention itself. This creates a challenge in distinguishing the program's impact from selection bias. Essentially, it's like conducting an experiment where participants select their own groups.

How can you tell if voluntary participation is hindering your transformation? Observe which departments regularly choose to join new initiatives and which consistently abstain. If the same divisions always opt out, you're not fostering widespread change—you're just deepening existing gaps. Consider whether non-participation has repercussions or is truly optional, with no accountability. Check whether transformation updates highlight the successes of "early adopters" while quietly ignoring those lagging. Honestly evaluate: after three years, has the gap between your top and bottom performers narrowed or expanded?

Voluntary efforts are ineffective. Without the authority to mandate necessary changes, transformation remains a luxury for the already best rather than driving comprehensive, system-wide progress.

THE UNCOMFORTABLE TRUTH

Voluntary transformation programs attract the people who need them least. The departments most in need of improvement are the ones most likely to opt out—and your leadership team lets them, because confrontation is uncomfortable. You're widening the gap between your best and worst performers while calling it "transformation."

. . .

KILLER #4: THE CEO MIRAGE

Every successful transformation depends on dedicated executive sponsorship. This is a consistent point made by all consultants and emphasized by every change management framework. It remains entirely true.

And it is entirely inadequate.

Here's what unfolds: An ambitious, visionary CEO steps in, bringing a history of successful transformation from their previous role. They are specifically hired to lead change within this organization. With strong board support, they initiate major projects, allocate resources, participate in meetings, and publicly champion the efforts. Their commitment is sincere.

After 18 to 36 months, they depart, whether due to recruitment by a larger institution, the board's impatience with progress, family relocation, or other reasons. The typical CEO tenure at academic medical centers is less than five years, but significant transformations generally take longer.

The new CEO brings their own vision, priorities, and consultants. The old initiatives are quietly set aside, and the transformation team is reassigned. Metrics are no longer monitored. In six months, it's as if the previous transformation never took place.

Over a decade, I've observed this cycle three times at a specific academic health system. CEO #1 initiated Lean transformation, CEO #2 shifted focus to High Reliability, and CEO #3 prioritized patient experience. All initiatives were well-planned and saw initial success. However, none persisted beyond leadership changes. The organization invested millions but failed to achieve lasting improvement.

The issue isn't a lack of commitment from the CEO, but rather reliance on it. When transformation relies solely on the CEO's support, it tends to falter once the CEO departs. Without embedding the change into structures—such as governance frameworks, budget processes, accountability systems, and cultural adjustments—initiatives that depend on the CEO's influence remain vulnerable.

How can you identify if CEO dependency poses a risk to your organization? Consider: if your current CEO announced they were leaving tomorrow, what impact would that have on your transformation efforts? Would those initiatives proceed smoothly, or would they become vulnerable? Assess how transformation is funded—are resources part of the regular operations budget or allocated as special project funds aligned with executive priorities? Review governance structures—are transformation initiatives integrated into permanent committees and decision-making processes, or are they treated as separate "special initiatives"? Also, observe whether frontline staff describe transformation as "the organization's work" or as "Dr. Smith's program."

If a transformation depends on individual leaders, it is destined to fail. Leadership changes are unavoidable in academic medicine. Your transformation must endure beyond these transitions.

KILLER #5: THE CULTURE DELUSION

Every unsuccessful transformation I've examined involved, at some point in the planning documents, references to "culture change." Leaders recognized that lasting transformation depends on a cultural shift. They noted that psychological safety, collaboration, and continuous learning must become ingrained as organizational standards.

Then, they attempted to alter culture using communication campaigns.

They produced posters highlighting "our values" and delivered speeches emphasizing "putting patients first." They used aspirational language to brand their transformation and shared success stories in newsletters. They believed that consistently articulating the desired culture would lead to a cultural shift.

It never happens that way. Culture evolves through structural change, not just communication.

I observed an academic medical center that invested eighteen months in a "culture transformation" initiative centered on psychological safety and blame-free learning. They held all-hands meetings, trained leaders in "appreciative inquiry," implemented feedback systems, and shared success stories. According to all communication metrics, the initiative was successful: 90% of staff could explain the new values, leaders consistently used appropriate language, and posters were displayed throughout the facility.

I interviewed frontline nurses about their sense of safety when raising patient safety concerns. One nurse summarized the disconnect well: "Sure, they say they want us to speak up. But when Dr. Johnson yells at you in front of the entire OR team, and nothing is done, you learn to stay silent. The posters don't make a difference."

Culture is demonstrated through what is tolerated, rewarded, or punished, not merely stated. It shows who is promoted, which behaviors lead to outcomes, how conflicts are resolved, the metrics that influence choices, and resource distribution. Without changing these structural elements, aspirational messages remain ineffective noise.

The harsh reality is that the governance structures responsible for your current culture are not capable of transforming it. Hierarchical decision-making fosters a hierarchical culture. Allocating resources competitively promotes a culture of competition. Focusing on individual performance metrics encourages individual-centric behavior. To cultivate a collaborative, learning-oriented culture, it is essential to implement structures that promote collaboration and learning.

How can you tell if you're attempting to drive culture change through communication rather than structural changes? Look for gaps between your stated values and actual outcomes. Check your promotion criteria—do they favor systems improvement or individual success? Review your budget process—does it foster collaboration or rivalry for resources? Consider your conflict resolution methods—are disagreements resolved through dialogue or hierarchy? Observe whether transformation meetings genuinely involve frontline staff as partners or are merely passive recipients of decisions. Honestly assess: when someone exemplifies the desired culture but threatens the existing power structure, who tends to win?

You can't resolve a structural issue through communication alone. Until the structure is altered, cultural change remains superficial.

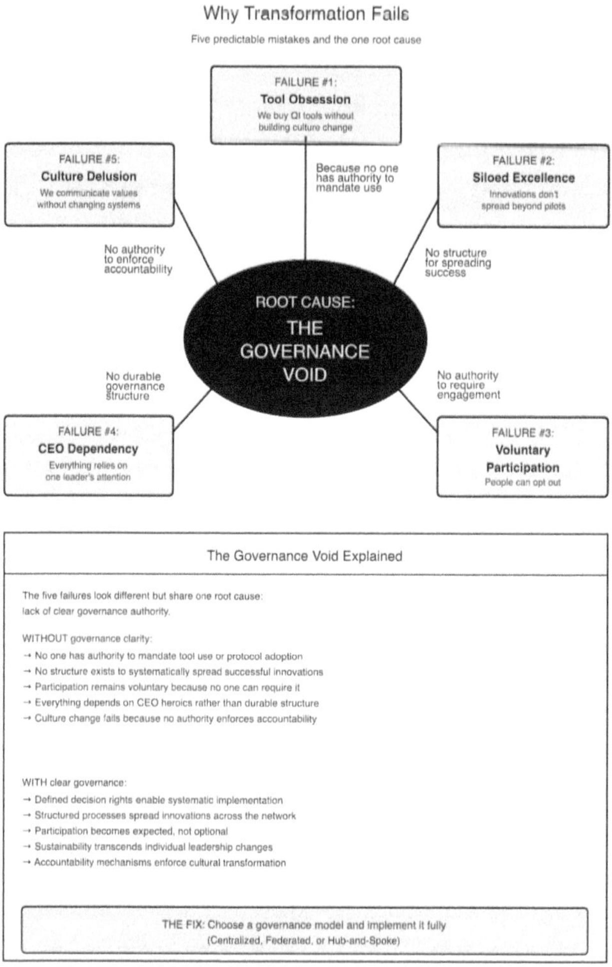

THE ROOT CAUSE: THE GOVERNANCE VOID

Five killers, each representing a different failure mode, all stem from a common root cause.

The governance void.

Academic health systems often overlook the fundamental question: Who truly decides? Who possesses the authority to enforce system-wide changes? Who can reassign resources from low-value to high-value activities? Who is responsible for holding departments accountable for overall system performance? And who has the power to eliminate ineffective initiatives?

I've repeated these questions many times, and the answers remain surprisingly consistent.

The dean of the medical school states, "I oversee medical education, but do not manage hospital operations."

The hospital COO states, "I oversee operations, but physicians are credentialed via the medical school."

Department chairs state, "We have clinical autonomy within our departments."

Community hospital presidents state, "We adopt practices that are best suited for our patient population."

Translation: No one can enforce improvement across the entire system. Everyone holds veto power. Nothing has ultimate authority.

This explains why tool obsession occurs—because promoting voluntary methods is simpler than enforcing mandatory change. It also clarifies why siloes continue—due to the absence of governance structures that compel collaboration. Participation remains voluntary—since no authority exists to require it. CEO transitions can be disastrous—because, without structural governance, outcomes rely heavily on personal influence. Finally, culture change often fails because the governance frameworks that shape culture have not been modified.

Without a clear governance—such as explicit decision rights, authority frameworks, and accountability systems—transformation cannot happen. It's not just challenging; it's impossible. You might have a flawless strategy, abundant resources, talented individuals, and full dedication. But without governance, your efforts are merely aspirations without the authority to implement them.

Academic health systems are especially susceptible to governance gaps due to their matrix structure. Faculty report to department chairs, who in turn report to deans. Clinicians deliver care in hospitals overseen by CEOs, whose influence over physician behavior varies. Research operates under distinct funding and governance structures. Accreditation standards and academic policies govern education. Including affiliated community hospitals with varying levels of autonomy creates a complex governance puzzle that would challenge any organization.

Many academic health systems address this by forming advisory committees that only recommend, task forces that analyze but cannot make decisions, and councils that gather but lack the power to enforce. These superficial governance structures create the illusion of coordination but lack real authority.

Genuine transformation demands genuine governance, not just advice or voluntary actions. It requires real authority to make decisions, allocate resources, and hold individuals accountable.

WHAT ACTUALLY WORKS

Let me show you what governance-first transformation looks like.

THE RIVERSIDE HEALTH SYSTEM STORY

Riverside Health System included a 600-bed academic medical center, a medical school, and seven community hospitals across three states. By 2019, they confronted a crisis: they were in the worst quartile nationally for 30-day readmissions, their patient safety culture scores had declined for three straight years, 68% of staff reported high burnout, and their operating margins were barely sustainable at 1.2%.

Leadership had exhausted all options. From 2015 to 2019, they implemented a Lean transformation with a $4.5M investment, engaged in High-Reliability Organization consulting, launched an "Always Events" patient experience program, formed physician wellness task forces, launched nurse retention initiatives, and undertook EHR optimization. Despite these efforts, no lasting results emerged. Staff became cynical, department chairs grew skeptical, and the board's patience waned.

In January 2020, the new CEO, Dr. Maria Chen, took charge. During her first 90 days, she asked consistently in every meeting: "Who has the authority to require us to adopt an evidence-based sepsis protocol across all eight hospitals?"

The answers highlighted the core issue: the medical school dean oversaw education but not hospital operations, while the hospital COO managed operations. Health regulators credentialed physicians, yet department chairs claimed clinical autonomy, and community hospital presidents implemented practices suited to their populations. Translation: no one could enforce system-wide improvements, as all had veto power, resulting in a lack of authority.

On day 91, Dr. Chen told the board: "Before we discuss strategy, we must address governance. Without clear decision-making authority, no strategy will succeed."

Dr. Chen advocated for clear decision rights. The Hub, an academic medical center, would create evidence-based protocols, train 25 quality improvement mentors across the system, enhance analytics skills, and assist with implementing spokes. The Spokes, comprising seven community hospitals, would tailor protocols locally, offer feedback to improve strategies, and share innovations.

The key point of controversy is that it should be a genuine authority rather than just another advisory committee. The System Learning Council would have direct control over a $3.5 million annual budget, the ability to mandate protocols when evidence warrants, the power to reallocate resources, and the authority to hold leaders accountable based on system metrics.

This meant some would lose autonomy. Department chairs would enforce system protocols. Community presidents would adopt hub approaches. The board approved it.

Phase 1 (Months 1-6): Hired a Chief Learning Officer, formed the System Learning Council, trained 25 QI mentors, created a baseline dashboard, and discontinued 11 out of 14 existing initiatives to decrease cognitive load.

Phase 2 (Months 7-12): Focused on five key system-wide priorities —sepsis mortality, hospital-acquired infections, 30-day readmissions, opioid stewardship, and staff psychological safety—rather than thirty. Each priority had dedicated hub teams and spoke implementation teams, with monthly learning calls and quarterly in-person meetings.

Phase 3 (Months 13-24): Expanded to eight priorities, trained an additional 20 mentors, launched peer mentoring, incorporated QI into residency curricula, and started publishing implementation insights.

Not everyone was pleased. Over the past 18 months, three department chairs have departed, seeking more autonomy than collaboration. A community hospital president who opposed hub protocols was replaced. Dr. Chen admitted, "We lost talented people. But we couldn't let individual preferences override system needs."

The three-year results reveal significant progress. Clinical quality saw a 34% reduction in hospital-acquired infections, a 28% decrease in sepsis mortality, a 19% decline in 30-day readmissions, and a 42% drop in central line infections. Culture metrics improved notably: patient safety scores rose 18 points, moving from the 40th to the 75th percentile nationally; physician burnout fell from 68% to 41%; nurse intent to leave decreased from 31% to 18%; staff engagement increased by 22 points. Financially, the operating margin expanded from 1.2% to 3.8%, with an 8% reduction in cost per case, leading to $4.2 million in annual savings from avoided HAI-related costs. The transformation's influence expanded: 45 QI mentors trained, 127 improvement projects completed, 23 peer-reviewed publications published, and the model adopted by three regional health systems.

Dr. Chen reflected, "I expected resistance. What surprised me was how rapidly things progressed once governance was clarified. Previously, every decision required consensus from 15 stakeholders—often involving meetings to plan other meetings—and it took 6 months to approve a pilot. Once governance was in place, decision-making shortened to weeks instead of months."

She mentioned, "If I had the chance to do it again, I would set up governance before my arrival. The initial 90 days were useful, but took a lot of time. If the board had finalized governance during the CEO search, we could have accelerated the process by six months."

Riverside's success was not due to superior consultants, resources, or more intelligent staff. Their victory stemmed from prioritizing governance first. All other aspects—such as protocols, training, mentoring, and measurement—were built upon that essential choice.

Lacking governance clarity leads to optional participation, whereas transparent governance drives transformation.

THE QUESTION

So here's the question for you.

Can you currently identify who in your organization has the authority to mandate system-wide clinical improvements? Who has the power to tell all departments, hospitals, and practices: "This is how we manage sepsis, and it must be followed"?

If you're unable to answer that question clearly and confidently, you've identified your core issue.

Until you resolve it, all transformation efforts—regardless of how well-intentioned, well-funded, or carefully designed—will become part of the majority that ultimately fail.

The good news is that you can resolve this issue. However, it involves making a choice that most academic health systems tend to avoid.

That decision—and how to make it—is what the next chapter is about.

BEFORE YOU CONTINUE

You've just read about five ways transformation efforts fail. Now apply them to yourself.

1. Of the five killers described in this chapter—tool obsession, siloed excellence, voluntary participation, CEO dependency, and the culture delusion—how many does your current or most recent transformation effort exhibit? If you answered fewer than three,

you're either extraordinarily lucky or not being honest with yourself.

2. Write down the name of the person in your organization who can mandate system-wide clinical improvements. Not "recommend" or "propose"—mandate. If you hesitated, couldn't think of anyone, or wrote down a committee name, you've just identified your core problem.

Name: ______________________________

3. Think of someone in your organization who has openly criticized your transformation efforts. Were they right? What happened to them? If critics are silenced, sidelined, or dismissed as "not team players," your organization punishes honest feedback—which means no one will tell you when transformation is failing until it's too late.

4. If your board approved "hub-and-spoke governance" tomorrow, what would actually happen when a department chair refused to adopt a mandated protocol? Would there be consequences? Who would enforce them? If you're uncertain, you don't have governance—you have governance theater.

5. You've now read about Riverside Health System's success. What's the first reason that came to mind for why their approach wouldn't work at your organization? Please write it down.

REASON: ______________________________

NOW ASK YOURSELF: Is that reason a genuine structural barrier, or is it the excuse you use to avoid difficult decisions? Most "reasons" are actually fear in disguise.

PART II

THE SOLUTION

3

THE GOVERNANCE DECISION

THREE VIABLE GOVERNANCE MODELS AND HOW TO CHOOSE THE RIGHT ONE FOR YOUR ORGANIZATION

THE QUESTION YOU'VE BEEN AVOIDING

The governance void isn't accidental; it's a deliberate choice—or rather, the lack of one. Academic health systems continually delay making this decision because it demands facing difficult truths about power, autonomy, and control.

Every academic health system leader I've collaborated with understands, in theory, that governance is important. They recognize that successful transformation depends on having clear authority. They have studied the change management literature and have heard consultants stress the importance of executive alignment.

Then they create governance frameworks that ensure no individual truly holds the authority to make decisions.

They establish steering committees that offer advice but lack the authority to enforce decisions. They set up task forces that suggest actions but cannot carry them out. They organize councils that deliberate without the power to compel. They create detailed governance diagrams illustrating reporting lines and dotted connections among stakeholders—complex organizational charts that accurately depict how decisions are ultimately not made.

Why? Granting someone or a group real authority over clinical practice, resource distribution, and performance standards across the system could disrupt the fragile power balance that sustains academic health systems. Department chairs might see their independence diminish. Medical school deans could relinquish control. Community hospital presidents might need to enforce protocols they didn't create. Faculty might be required to cooperate instead of compete.

Rather than addressing the issue head-on, most organizations engage in governance theater. They present the appearance of coordination without genuinely granting the authority needed to coordinate effectively.

Here's what I need you to realize: avoiding this decision isn't possible; the only option is to delay it. Each month you put it off, another month your transformation efforts are at risk of failure.

The good news is that there are three viable governance models available. All of them are effective and have been successfully implemented in various academic health systems. Each model can drive transformation successfully—provided you commit to it wholeheartedly and execute it with honesty.

The unfortunate reality is that you must make a choice. You can't merge the options into a balanced compromise that respects everyone's independence. Keeping your options open doesn't work as a hedge. Unclear governance is more problematic than any imperfect but fully implemented model.

Let me present the three models, explaining what they offer, their costs, and how to select among them.

THE UNCOMFORTABLE TRUTH

You don't have a governance problem because you haven't figured out the right model. You have a governance problem because the right model requires people—possibly including you—to give up autonomy they don't want to give up. The intellectual challenge is trivial; the political challenge is enormous.

. . .

THE THREE GOVERNANCE MODELS

Every successful learning organization transformation I've examined employs one of three governance models: Centralized, Federated, or Hub-and-Spoke. These models go beyond simple organizational charts; they represent fundamentally different methods for decision-making, knowledge sharing, and determining authority.

Before I discuss each model, keep in mind: the question isn't "which model is best?" but rather "which model fits our organizational reality and strategic priorities?" A model that performs well at one institution may fail at another—not due to a flaw in the model but because it doesn't suit the specific context.

The three models span from full central control to complete local autonomy. Your task is to identify the optimal balance point on this spectrum that harmonizes your desire for consistency with your need for flexibility. Making the wrong choice could either suppress local innovation through strict standardization or cause fragmentation by granting too much autonomy.

Let me walk you through each model.

MODEL ONE: CENTRALIZED - CONTROL FIRST

The centralized model places decision-making authority mainly at the system level, usually at the leading academic medical center. System leadership defines policies, protocols, and performance standards that affiliated sites are expected to follow accurately. Knowledge mainly flows from the center outward. Compliance with these standards is regularly monitored and enforced diligently.

This model is effective when maintaining consistency and standardization across the network is your top priority. Centralized governance ensures compliance with regulations, patient safety standards, and technology integration across the entire organization. It also enables quick, system-wide adoption of evidence-based practices through authoritative mandates. Additionally, if your organization aims to project a unified identity to external stakeholders, centralization provides clear, consistent messaging.

I observed this model succeed at a mid-sized academic health system in the Southwest. Their new CEO, a physician with extensive quality improvement expertise, inherited an organization with significant performance variation across units. Sepsis mortality rates ranged from 12% to 28% among different departments. Hospital-acquired infection rates varied by a factor of three. Patient safety culture scores ranged from the 25th to the 85th percentile. This variation wasn't due to patient acuity or case mix; it depended on the specific department.

The CEO established strict centralized governance, providing extensive PDSA and systems thinking training to all clinical directors and department heads. Daily leadership huddles monitored key metrics and identified barriers. The CEO personally conducted daily gemba walks, observing workflows and engaging with staff through questions. A system-wide balanced scorecard offered real-time performance visibility to everyone. Most crucially, adherence to evidence-based protocols became mandatory. Department chairs resisting compliance faced a direct choice: follow the protocols or relinquish their leadership roles.

Within eighteen months, the outcomes were impressive: medication errors decreased by 45%, emergency department wait times reduced by 35%, patient satisfaction scores rose to the top decile nationwide, staff engagement increased by 28%, and financial margins improved due to efficiency gains—highlighted by the emergency department redesign that saved $2M annually in operational costs.

However, centralized governance has significant drawbacks. It can suppress local innovation if a single approach is mandated from the top. Solutions that are not suitable for local contexts may be enforced anyway. Frontline staff might feel ignored when decisions are made at the system level without their involvement. This model is most effective when central leadership possesses exceptional expertise and when standardization offers real value. It performs poorly when central leaders are detached from local conditions or when standardization leads to generic solutions that fail to meet specific needs.

The centralized model requires exceptional leadership. When all decisions go through a central authority, the quality of that leadership determines the organization's overall performance. Visionary and capable central leaders promote excellence, while weak leaders cause bottlenecks and poor decisions that affect the entire system. Additionally, when strong central leaders depart, the organization becomes vulnerable unless their successors possess similar skills and dedication.

Opt for centralized governance when maintaining consistency is more important than local customization, especially if you have strong central leadership. Consider this approach if your organization needs urgent standardization and you're prepared for the possibility that some talented individuals who prioritize autonomy over collaboration may depart.

MODEL TWO: FEDERATED - SPEED WITH GUARDRAILS

The federated model grants significant autonomy to individual sites or regions while setting system-level guardrails, such as minimum standards, shared values, and core policies that everyone must follow. Each entity customizes central frameworks to fit its local context, makes most operational decisions independently, and innovates based on local needs. Knowledge sharing happens both horizontally among peers and vertically from system leadership.

This model is effective when speed and local relevance are your main concerns. If your organization operates across multiple geographic markets with distinct patient populations and competitive environments, granting local teams autonomy enables quick adaptation to local circumstances. To promote experimentation and innovation, decentralizing decision-making fosters creativity. When serving diverse communities with unique needs, local customization delivers better results than uniform strategies.

I observed the federated model succeed at a major academic medical center with a strong research culture. They chose to embrace their academic strengths rather than resist them. The School of Medicine integrated quality improvement scholarship into the medical student curriculum, requiring all students to complete QI projects for graduation. They also built a hospital-wide improvement network in which various clinical departments focused on locally identified priorities within system guidelines. Additionally, they created a research center dedicated to implementation science, transforming their efforts into publishable research.

Innovation thrived, with 48 improvement projects in their first year, covering clinical quality, education, and research transfer. Clinical outcomes showed improvements in various areas. The organization published 15 peer-reviewed papers about their implementation efforts. It gained global recognition as a learning organization. Residents trained there adopted the learning organization approach and spread it to other institutions, helping the model grow naturally.

However, the federated model introduces several significant challenges. Coordination among independent initiatives is complex, and quality and outcomes often vary widely across sites—some departments adopt learning organization principles, while others show minimal engagement. Without effective central coordination, organizations risk duplicating efforts as sites independently tackle similar issues. Implementing system-wide changes becomes more complicated when each site has the autonomy to opt out. Additionally, research-oriented cultures occasionally prioritize publishing over real-world impact, focusing more on studying transformation than actually accomplishing it.

A successful federated model relies on advanced infrastructure. This includes strong communities of practice that facilitate peer learning, clear guardrails setting minimum standards while allowing local flexibility, and knowledge sharing platforms to disseminate innovations across sites. System leadership should prioritize convening, connecting, and synthesizing rather than exerting control.

Without such infrastructure, federated governance risks fragmentation.

Opt for federated governance when operating across diverse markets that need local adaptation, fostering innovation and experimentation. This approach is suitable if your sites have strong leadership capable of making independent decisions, your culture promotes academic freedom and intellectual pursuit, and you're open to variations in methods and results in exchange for local innovation.

MODEL THREE: HUB-AND-SPOKE - BALANCING CONTROL AND OUTCOMES

The hub-and-spoke model assigns a central academic medical center as the hub, which offers specialized services, advanced expertise, protocol development, training, and mentorship. Community hospitals and clinics serve as spokes, providing routine care, applying hub-developed protocols tailored to their local context, and offering feedback to improve system approaches. Authority is distributed, with responsibilities clearly defined between the hub and spokes.

This is the model Riverside Health System adopted, as described in Chapter 2. The hub developed evidence-based protocols in collaboration with multidisciplinary teams and trained QI mentors across the system. The spokes applied these protocols with local adaptations and offered real-world feedback. The System Learning Council—equipped with genuine budget authority and decision-making power—decided when standardization was necessary and when local variation was permissible.

The hub-and-spoke model works effectively when both centralized coordination and local responsiveness are required. A robust central academic medical center with extensive expertise acts as a resource multiplier across the network. Meanwhile, community hospitals and clinics serving diverse populations benefit from spoke autonomy, allowing for contextual adaptation. This model also facilitates bidirectional knowledge transfer: systematic sharing from the hub to the spokes and practice-based learning from the spokes back to the hub.

This model maintains consistency in core standards while permitting local customization. It effectively leverages central expertise across the network rather than expecting every site to develop all capabilities independently. It establishes clear channels for knowledge sharing, such as mentoring programs, learning collaboratives, and communities of practice. This approach strikes a balance between efficiency and responsiveness, allowing for standardization where beneficial and customization as necessary.

However, hub-and-spoke governance demands substantial investment in coordination infrastructure. This includes establishing systematic processes for protocol development at the hub and providing implementation support for spokes. Mentoring relationships between hub experts and spoke teams are essential. Regular meetings should facilitate collective reflection and ongoing improvement. Clear role definitions are necessary so that everyone understands the responsibilities and decision-making rights of both hub and spokes. Importantly, genuine partnership is crucial—spoke voices should actively influence hub decisions, rather than merely following hub mandates.

The model breaks down when the hub lacks sufficient expertise or capacity to perform its role. It also fails when spokes perceive themselves as subordinates instead of partners. Additionally, it struggles when the coordination infrastructure is underfunded or underdeveloped. Moreover, it encounters difficulties when hub-and-spoke leaders cannot agree on the right balance between standardization and local adaptation.

Opt for hub-and-spoke governance if you have a strong academic medical center that can act as a capability hub, especially when you require both system-wide consistency and local adaptability. This structure is suitable if you are willing to invest in coordination infrastructure and mentorship, and if you prioritize bidirectional knowledge exchange over top-down control. Additionally, it works best when both hub and spoke leaders are prepared to share authority and responsibility.

THE DECISION POINT

You're the CEO of a 400-bed academic medical center. Your CMO has developed an evidence-based sepsis protocol that reduced mortality by 28% in pilot units. You want to mandate it system-wide.

Dr. Martinez, chair of Surgery and your highest-revenue generator, refuses to adopt it. "My team has been managing sepsis for twenty years," he says. "We don't need a protocol designed by hospitalists telling us what to do."

Your board has approved hub-and-spoke governance, but Dr. Martinez is politically powerful, well-connected to board members, and his departure would cost you $4M in annual revenue.

WHAT DO YOU DO?

If you answered "find a compromise" or "give him time to come around," ask yourself: How is that different from what you've always done? How many patients will suffer while you wait for Dr. Martinez to change voluntarily?

If you answered "enforce the protocol regardless," ask yourself: Are you actually willing to do this? What happens when Dr. Martinez complains to his board contacts? Do you have your board's genuine support for enforcement, or just their theoretical approval?

This scenario isn't hypothetical. Some version of it happens at every academic health system attempting transformation. Your answer reveals whether you have genuine governance or governance theater.

What I would actually do: ______________________________

____

Three Governance Models: Comparison Matrix

Choose the model that aligns with your organizational priorities

DIMENSION	CENTRALIZED (Control First)	FEDERATED (Speed + Guardrails)	HUB-AND-SPOKE (Balanced)
Decision Rights	System leadership makes decisions; sites implement	Sites decide within system guardrails	Shared: Hub develops, spokes adapt locally
When to Use	· Consistency is paramount · Safety/regulatory requirements · Strong central expertise	· Speed and local fit are critical · Diverse markets · Innovation focus · Strong site leaders	· Need both control and responsiveness · Academic health systems (typical) · Hub has expertise
Key Strengths	· Rapid system-wide standardization · Clear accountability · Economies of scale · Unified brand identity	· Local innovation · Context-specific solutions · High staff engagement · Multiple solutions	· Core consistency + local adaptation · Leverage central expertise broadly · Bidirectional learning
Key Limitations	· One-size-fits-all solutions · Stifles local innovation · Slow local response · Central bottlenecks	· Quality variation across sites · Duplicated effort · Fragmentation risk · Difficult system-wide change	· Requires heavy coordination · Hub dominance risk · Role clarity essential
Resource Investment	Strong central capability + change management	Collaboration infrastructure + coordination	Mentoring network + bidirectional communication
Knowledge Flow	**Center → Sites**	**Site ↔ Site**	**Hub ↔ Spokes**

See Chapter 3 for detailed decision framework and implementation guidance.

HOW TO CHOOSE: THE DECISION FRAMEWORK

Select a governance model that aligns with three key factors: your strategic priorities, your organizational context, and your leadership capabilities.

Begin by identifying your organization's strategic priorities. What is most critical at this moment? If ensuring compliance and uniformity is essential—especially when you're under regulatory pressure or facing safety issues that demand rapid standardization—centralized governance is advisable. Conversely, if agility and local customization are more important—such as in competitive, diverse markets or innovation-focused environments—federated governance might be preferable. For situations requiring both control and flexibility—keeping core practices consistent while allowing local adaptations—a hub-and-spoke model could be the best fit.

Your organizational context influences what is possible. Consider how geographically spread out you are. Organizations across multiple states or regions might find centralized governance challenging, especially when frequent in-person coordination is needed. Reflect on the cultural diversity of your sites. Academic medical centers often have different cultures than community hospitals, so centralizing all functions could face resistance. Also, consider your history. Organizations with a tradition of departmental autonomy might resist rapid centralization, whereas those with a record of successful system-wide initiatives may be more open to it.

Leadership capabilities define what you can implement. Centralized structures require strong central leadership with extensive expertise and change-management skills. Federated setups require capable site leaders who can make independent decisions, along with system leaders adept at bringing people together and building connections. Hub-and-spoke arrangements require both hub knowledge and spoke leadership, as well as investment in mentoring infrastructure. Select a model aligned with your current leadership capacity, not just your aspirational goals.

Also consider resource availability. Centralized models can reduce duplication but require strong central capabilities and change-management resources. Federated models require collaboration infrastructure and coordination resources. Hub-and-spoke models demand investment in mentoring relationships and two-way communication. Make sure you can properly resource the model you select.

Another critical point is that governance models can change over time. Some organizations start with a centralized approach to establish standard practices, then move toward a federated or hub-and-spoke model as local capabilities develop. Others initially adopt a federated model and later centralize certain functions based on their experience. Hybrid models are also possible—such as having patient safety and regulatory compliance managed centrally. At the same time, clinical quality improvement uses a hub-and-spoke approach, and community health programs operate in a federated manner. The crucial aspect is clarity: clearly specify which governance model applies to each domain.

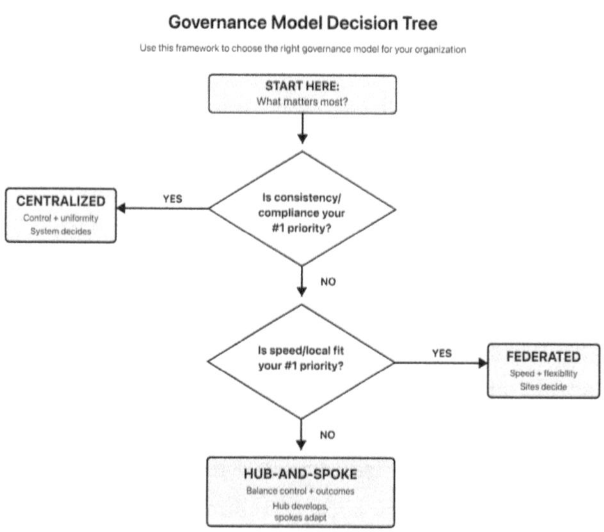

THE CONVERSATION YOU NEED TO HAVE

Practically speaking, your upcoming board, executive, or strategic planning meeting should have a clear agenda item: choosing a governance model for developing a learning organization.

Come prepared to discuss your core strategic priorities—are they consistency, speed, or both? Consider your organizational context, including geographic spread, cultural diversity, and resource availability. Also, assess your current leadership capabilities—not just aspirationally but in the present. Finally, determine which governance model best aligns with these realities.

Make the decision clear, document it, communicate it widely, and act on it completely. A solid governance model that's fully executed is better than a brilliant one that's half-hearted. Either commit fully or don't, but avoid wavering.

One last caution: the typical mistake is selecting a model without truly executing it. Boards often approve hub-and-spoke governance but fail to grant the System Learning Council meaningful budgetary authority. Executives might declare centralized governance yet allow departments to opt out if they oppose it. Leaders support federated governance but often neglect to invest in the necessary coordination infrastructure.

If you're selecting a governance model, make sure it's genuine. Provide it with authority, real resources, and accountability. Avoid creating superficial governance structures that offer only advice, without the power to enforce decisions.

The change you seek depends on having the authority to implement it. This is what governance provides—if you're honest about power, transparent in decision-making, and dedicated to accountability.

Now you know the models. You understand the decision framework. You see what success looks like.

The question is whether you're ready to make the choice.

Because the next step—the first 90 days of implementation—depends entirely on having governance clarity before you begin.

That's what the next Chapter is about.

BEFORE YOU CONTINUE

The governance decision isn't an intellectual exercise. It's a commitment. Before you proceed to implementation, answer these questions.

1. Which governance model fits your organization? Please write it down. If you wrote "hybrid" or "it depends," you're avoiding the decision. Every hybrid model is really one model with exceptions—so which is your primary model?

Primary governance model: ______________________________

2. Who will lose power or autonomy if you implement this model? Name them specifically. If you can't name anyone, your governance model probably doesn't change anything meaningful.

Names: ____

3. What will you do when the first influential person refuses to comply with a governance decision they disagree with? Not what you hope will happen—what will you actually do? If your answer involves "having a conversation" or "building consensus," you haven't committed to genuine governance.

4. Have you personally discussed this governance model with your board chair and received explicit support for enforcement authority? If not, schedule that conversation before reading further. Reading the next chapter without board alignment is a waste of time.

5. On a scale of 1-10, how committed are you—personally—to implementing this governance model even if it means losing talented people who prefer autonomy over collaboration? Be honest. If your number is below 7, you're not ready.

YOUR COMMITMENT LEVEL: _____ / 10

4

THE FIRST 90 DAYS

WEEK-BY-WEEK GUIDANCE FOR ESTABLISHING GENUINE FOUNDATION INSTEAD OF TRANSFORMATION THEATER

DAY ONE

You've finalized the governance decision and selected your model—whether centralized, federated, or hub-and-spoke. The board has given its approval, and the organization is aware that transformation is on the horizon.

Now what?

This is often where most transformation efforts fail early on. Leaders believe that once a strategic decision is made, implementation will automatically follow. They announce the transformation, set up a steering committee, possibly hire a consultant, and expect progress to begin.

Three months on, little has changed. Activities like meetings, presentations, and consultant payments have occurred, but there is no real transformation, measurable progress, or fundamental change in the organization's operations.

The issue isn't a shortage of commitment or resources. Instead, the first 90 days weren't utilized strategically; they were filled with activity that seemed productive but didn't genuinely lay the groundwork for transformation.

Let me demonstrate what the first 90 days should realistically entail. Not just hopeful ideas or theories, but what you genuinely need to achieve, step by step, to ensure your transformation has the best chance of success.

These 90 days will determine whether your transformation succeeds or becomes another failure. Please make the most of them.

WEEKS 1-2: CONFIRM GOVERNANCE ISN'T THEATER

I know you just spent the previous Chapter making the governance decision. The board approved it. You're ready to move forward.

Not so fast.

Here's what I've observed: Boards often approve governance models without fully understanding their implications. When they hear terms like "hub-and-spoke governance," it sounds reasonable, and they tend to approve it. However, about six months later, when the System Learning Council moves to enforce a protocol over departmental objections, board members start questioning their approval. They ask, "Wait, I didn't realize we were compromising clinical autonomy," or, "I thought this was meant to be collaborative, not merely directive," and, "Did we actually authorize budget reallocations without explicit board approval?"

The governance you believed you had disappears the first time you attempt to use it.

In the first two weeks, you need to verify that governance is genuine and not just symbolic. This involves having clear and sometimes challenging discussions about the true nature of authority.

Schedule one-on-one meetings with each board member and each member of your executive leadership team. These should be individual conversations, not group sessions, to encourage honest feedback without peer pressure. Ask everyone the same questions: "When I mentioned implementing hub-and-spoke governance, what was your understanding? What decisions do you believe the System Learning Council can make independently? If the council mandates a sepsis protocol and the Surgery chair refuses to follow it, what are the consequences? Who has the authority to act?"

Pay close attention to the answers. You're not aiming for perfect agreement, but rather to identify core misunderstandings that could cause issues later. Suppose the board chair views the System Learning Council as merely advisory, while you believe it has mandate authority. In that case, this is a problem to address now—not after six months when you attempt to exercise that authority.

Document what you hear. If several board members share the same concern or confusion, it's a sign to clarify governance explicitly before moving forward. Investing two weeks to achieve proper alignment is better than spending six months building on a shaky foundation of misunderstanding.

By the end of week two, ensure everyone understands and supports the governance model, or identifies concerns that need to be addressed. If there's fundamental misalignment, pause and clarify with the board. Avoid proceeding with unclear governance, as it will lead to failure.

Over the next two weeks, start forming your core implementation team. Include a project director or chief learning officer to oversee daily activities. Ensure you have executive sponsorship from the CEO or the person responsible for transformation. Gather representatives from key stakeholder groups, including clinical leadership, quality improvement, IT, education, and frontline staff. Keep the team small, ideally between eight and twelve members, as larger groups can be challenging to manage.

Hold your initial core team meeting by the end of the second week. The agenda should include reviewing the governance model, clarifying decision rights, setting the meeting schedule, and assigning initial responsibilities. This team will serve as the operational driver of your transformation, so it's important to invest effort in doing it correctly.

THE UNCOMFORTABLE TRUTH

The governance your board approved and the governance they'll actually support when tested are often different things. Board members approve "hub-and-spoke governance" without understanding it means someone will lose autonomy. Test their commitment now, before you build on a foundation of misunderstanding.

WEEKS 3-4: ASSESS REALITY HONESTLY

You've established governance and assembled your core team. Next, it's essential to assess your initial position with absolute honesty.

Most organizational assessments are often ineffective. They tend to boost leaders' confidence rather than uncover the truth. Consultants usually hesitate to highlight severe dysfunctions, fearing it will cost them clients. Internal teams might downplay issues to avoid appearing negative or disloyal. As a result, assessments are usually softened, problems are minimized, and organizations move forward with transformations based on illusions instead of facts.

Your evaluation should be honest and unflinching, even if the truth is uncomfortable.

Utilize a structured readiness framework, such as the seven-dimension model that includes leadership commitment, organizational culture, data infrastructure, quality improvement capacity, communication systems, resources, and the external environment. However, avoid merely distributing surveys and compiling scores. Instead, integrate quantitative survey data with qualitative interviews and direct observations for a more comprehensive assessment.

Interview fifteen to twenty opinion leaders within your organization—individuals who will be honest because they have credibility to protect. Ask them: "If we announced tomorrow that all departments must adopt a system-wide sepsis protocol, what would actually happen? Who would implement it right away? Who would resist?

Why?" Their responses will give you a more accurate picture of your actual preparedness than any survey score.

Observe real meetings and workflows instead of relying solely on what people say about their culture. Attend a department quality improvement meeting to see how team members respond when concerns are raised. Do they show curiosity or defensiveness? Do junior staff speak openly or defer to hierarchy? These observations reveal whether genuine psychological safety exists or if it's merely aspirational language in your values statement.

Evaluate your data systems critically. Are you able to extract the necessary data to assess progress? How quickly can you generate a performance report? What is the quality of your data? I've seen organizations start ambitious improvement projects only to realize, after six months, that they cannot determine whether there has been any improvement because their data systems fail to provide reliable metrics.

By the end of week four, you should have a detailed assessment of your organization's readiness across all significant areas. Identify and document strengths to leverage and gaps to address. Be specific: avoid vague statements like "culture needs work" and instead say, "staff in three of five departments report they do not feel safe raising concerns about physician behavior." Similarly, rather than "data systems need improvement," specify, "the current EHR setup cannot track sepsis bundle compliance; fixing this would take six months and cost $200K."

Share this assessment with your board and executive team. Some may feel uneasy with the honesty, but that's acceptable—being uncomfortable with truth is preferable to being deluded. If your assessment shows you're not yet prepared for transformation, delay it until you address your core gaps. Starting a transformation without solid readiness is like constructing a house on sand—an impressive attempt that is doomed to fail.

THE UNCOMFORTABLE TRUTH

If your readiness assessment doesn't identify significant problems, it wasn't honest. No organization is ready for transformation in all dimensions. An assessment that says "we're basically ready" is an assessment designed to confirm what leadership wanted to hear.

WEEKS 5-8: DEVELOP VISION THROUGH DIALOGUE

You have clarity on governance and understand your readiness. The next step is to develop a shared vision—an inspiring and compelling picture of what success looks like that motivates commitment, not just compliance.

Most organizational visions are often formed incorrectly. Usually, senior leaders go on a retreat, develop an aspirational statement, reveal it to the organization, and expect everyone to support it. However, the result is usually polite agreement followed by disengagement. Employees don't genuinely commit to visions imposed on them; they are more committed to those they help develop.

Developing a vision should be a four-week dialogue involving diverse stakeholders at various levels. Begin with board and executive leaders, not to craft the vision but to discuss the key questions it must address: What problems are we aiming to solve? What does success look like for patients, clinicians, our community, and our academic mission? What sacrifices are we prepared to make to reach this goal? What makes this worthwhile despite the challenges of transformation?

These initial discussions highlight tensions that must be openly acknowledged. Board members often focus on financial sustainability, while clinical leaders emphasize quality improvement, and educators focus on integrating the academic mission. The vision should address all these aspects—not by ignoring the tensions, but by explaining how developing a learning organization can support multiple goals at once.

Following executive alignment, hold visioning sessions with a broader range of stakeholders. Invite department chairs, clinical leaders, frontline staff, patient representatives, and community partners. Use structured facilitation to explore their goals and aspirations. Ask what they hope the transformation will achieve, what frustrations they want to see resolved, and what opportunities they identify.

Identify recurring themes across groups. If nurses, physicians, and administrators all highlight the same frustrations—such as fragmented communication, duplicated efforts, or challenges in maintaining improvements—your vision should focus on these. Similarly, when both patients and clinicians express a desire for more time for genuine conversations over merely completing checklists, it signals a vital area for attention.

Create a draft vision statement based on what you hear, capturing stakeholders' genuine aspirations rather than generic consultant-speak. Effective vision statements should be specific enough to inform decisions, ambitious enough to motivate action, and authentic enough to reflect people's values.

Test the draft vision with the same stakeholder groups by asking: "Does this reflect what you told us? Does this inspire your commitment? Does this guide decisions about priorities?" Refine it based on their feedback. Although this iterative process takes time—four weeks may seem slow when a rapid transformation is needed—creating a vision through dialogue fosters commitment that speeds up subsequent steps. Conversely, a vision imposed from the top fosters compliance but can weaken overall progress.

By the end of week eight, you should have a vision statement that the board has approved, with executive leadership champions and broader stakeholder groups viewing it as a true reflection of their goals. This vision then serves as your North Star throughout the entire transformation.

WEEKS 9-12: DESIGN QUICK WINS STRATEGICALLY

You have governance, a readiness assessment, and a shared vision. You're prepared to begin actual improvement efforts, but not with large-scale initiatives that take years to show results. Instead, focus on strategic quick wins that can demonstrate value within 90 days.

Quick wins are essential for three reasons. First, they boost stakeholder confidence, showing that transformation can happen in practice, not just in theory. Second, they help create early advocates—those who see improvements firsthand become your supporters. Third, they help build momentum and political support, which are essential for addressing more difficult, long-term changes.

However, quick wins should be selected strategically rather than opportunistically. The temptation might be to focus on easy problems that can be solved quickly, even if they lack significance. Avoid this approach. Quick wins that do not align with strategic priorities can squander your early-mover advantage.

Use three criteria to identify quick wins: high visibility, meaning people notice the improvement; precise measurement, allowing impact demonstration with data within 90 days; and strategic alignment, ensuring the initiative supports your priorities.

Between weeks nine and twelve, pinpoint three to five quick wins that meet these criteria. For each, perform a quick assessment: determine the current situation, identify improvement opportunities, consider potential interventions, define success, establish measurement methods, and assign a leader.

Involve frontline staff in pinpointing quick wins, as they understand which issues can be easily solved and which are more challenging. They are aware of improvements that could make their tasks more straightforward or more difficult. Their ideas often go unheard because no one seeks their input. For example, frontline nurses might say, "We waste fifteen minutes every shift searching for equipment—if we had standardized locations, we could save hours," which represents a clear opportunity for quick improvement.

Choose two or three quick wins to implement right away—nothing more. Focus on a few initiatives that can quickly show tangible results, rather than spreading effort thin across many. Clearly assign leadership, set a 90-day timeline to achieve measurable progress, and define success metrics.

Also, from weeks nine to twelve, prepare your organization for the transformation launch by developing a communication plan that explains what's coming and why. Create a stakeholder engagement plan to ensure ongoing involvement. Establish baseline metrics to track progress. Establish governance structures and meeting schedules to ensure the operational infrastructure is in place.

By day ninety, you'll be ready to confidently announce your transformation. You will have governance clarity, an honest assessment, a shared vision, and already in progress, quick wins. This isn't about announcing aspirations—it's about presenting tangible evidence of progress.

> THE UNCOMFORTABLE TRUTH
>
> Quick wins are necessary but dangerous. They build momentum—but they also create the temptation to declare success too early. The real test of transformation isn't whether you can win quickly, but whether you can sustain wins over the years. Anyone can improve a metric for 90 days.

THE DECISION POINT

Your transformation team has identified two potential quick wins:

Option A: A medication reconciliation improvement in the Cardiology unit. The team is enthusiastic, the chair is supportive, and early metrics show a 40% improvement in the pilot. Cardiology is already one of your highest-performing departments.

Option B: A hand hygiene compliance initiative in General Surgery, where compliance rates have been stubbornly low for years. The surgical chair is skeptical, the team is resistant, but infection rates are a serious patient safety issue.

Option A will almost certainly succeed and generate positive publicity. Option B might fail, and even if it succeeds, the surgical chair might undermine your credibility.

Which do you choose?

If you chose Option A, you're playing it safe—building momentum with a willing department while avoiding the more complex challenge. This is a reasonable choice, but be honest about what you're doing: you're strengthening the strong, not the weak.

If you choose Option B, you're taking a risk that could undermine early momentum if it fails. But you're also demonstrating that transformation isn't voluntary and that patient safety matters more than political comfort.

There's no obviously correct answer. But be honest about the trade-offs. Most organizations default to Option A and then wonder why their transformation only reaches departments that were already performing well.

My choice and my reasoning: ________________________

____

WHAT HAPPENS ON DAY 91

Day ninety-one marks the point when transformation is announced to the whole organization: "We're transforming into a learning organization. Here's what that entails. Why it matters. What we've achieved in the first 90 days. And what's next?"

You highlight existing governance structures that are already in place and functional. You share the results of the readiness assessment, including both strengths and areas for improvement. You present the shared vision developed with stakeholders. You showcase early successes that are already yielding results. You outline the next steps along with practical timelines.

This announcement is credible because you spent 90 days laying the foundation. You're not just selling hope; you're showing progress.

Most organizations start incorrectly. They announce a transformation with much fanfare on the first day, then spend months figuring out the details. Stakeholders see the chaos, become cynical, and disconnect. Instead, focus on doing the hard work first, then communicate once you're ready with concrete results.

After day ninety, your focus moves from establishing the foundation to actively implementing your plans. If you selected hub-and-spoke governance, you start engaging spoke sites. You also initiate additional improvement projects that build on quick win successes. Furthermore, you set up systematic learning cycles—monthly metric reviews, quarterly stakeholder feedback, and ongoing adjustments based on insights gained.

However, none of these efforts are effective without the foundation built in the first 90 days. Without clarity, governance becomes mere theater. Assessment driven by dishonesty fosters delusion. Vision advanced without dialogue meets resistance. Implementation that misses quick wins risks losing momentum.

The first 90 days aren't just about preparing for transformation; they are the transformation itself—the essential groundwork that decides the success of everything that follows.

You've now completed three chapters that explain why transformation often fails, how to select an appropriate governance model, and how to make the most of your first 90 days. At this point, you're transparent about the actions needed and their timing.

The question is whether you'll actually do it.

The next chapter, which covers the three essential capabilities you need to develop, assumes you have established this foundation. Without it, your capability development is likely to fail, just as other efforts have.

Let me show you what those capabilities are and why they're non-negotiable.

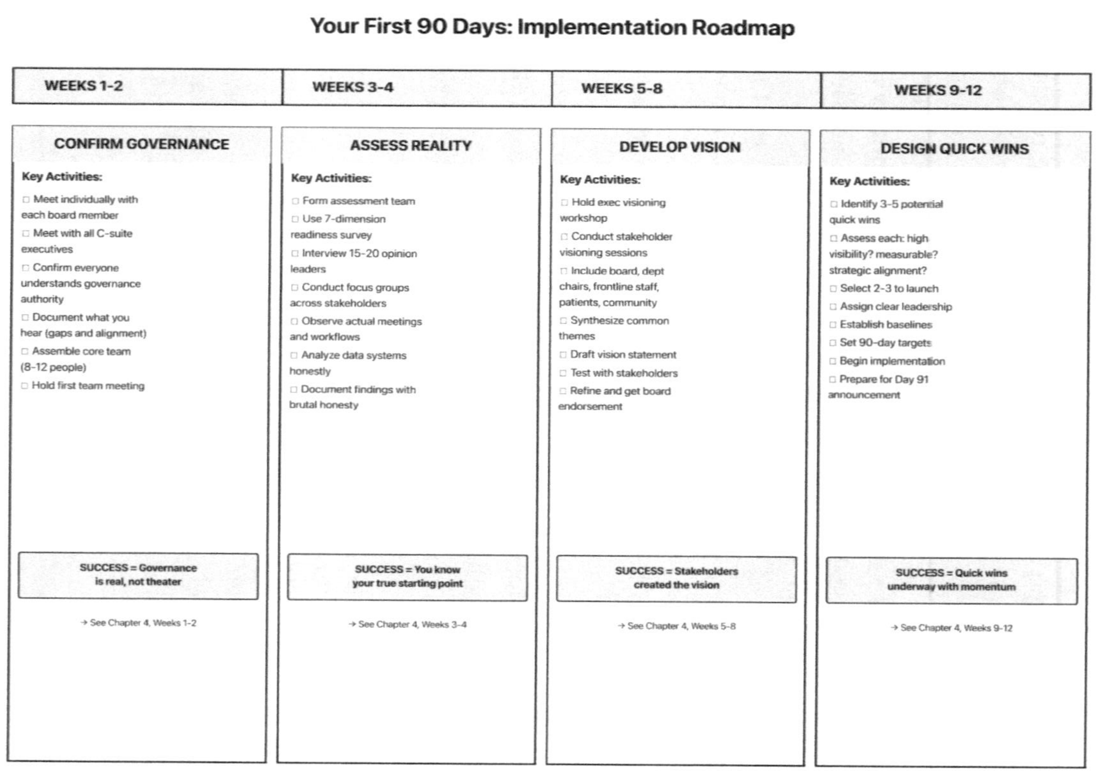

Figure 3: The First 90 Days Implementation Roadmap (See Chapter 4 for complete guidance)

BEFORE YOU CONTINUE

You now have a 90-day roadmap. But roadmaps don't implement themselves.

1. What date is 90 days from today? Write it here. This is your target date for completing Phase 1. If you can't commit to a specific date, you're not ready to start.

Date 90 days from now: ____________________

2. Who will lead the governance confirmation conversations in Weeks 1-2? This person needs authority, political skill, and willingness to hear uncomfortable truths. If you're thinking "I should probably do it myself," ask whether you have time and whether you're the right person to hear honest feedback about governance gaps.

Person responsible: ____________________

3. What will you stop doing to free up time for transformation initiatives? The roadmap demands considerable leadership focus. If you try to add this to your existing commitments, success becomes unlikely. Identify three tasks you can deprioritize, delegate, or remove.

I will stop/reduce:

a. ____________________

b. ____________________

c. ____________________

4. During Weeks 3-4 readiness assessment, what finding would delay the transformation? Which gap is critical enough to postpone instead of proceeding? If you say "nothing—we're committed," then you're not really assessing but just going through the motions.

5. Who will honestly inform you if your first 90 days go poorly? Not just your direct reports—who has the courage and credibility to deliver bad news? Identify them. If you can't name someone who can tell you when things are off track, your transformation may be at risk.

My honest feedback source: ____________________

5

THE THREE ESSENTIAL CAPABILITIES

BUILDING PSYCHOLOGICAL SAFETY, QI MENTORING NETWORKS, AND DATA-DRIVEN LEARNING CYCLES

THE INFRASTRUCTURE QUESTION

You've built the foundation. You have clarity of governance, honest assessment, a shared vision, and early momentum from strategic quick wins. Your organization is ready to scale transformation beyond pilot projects and early adopters.

Now you face the infrastructure question: What organizational capabilities must you build to enable sustained learning across your entire system?

This is where most academic health systems make a critical error. They assume that if they train enough people in quality improvement methods, provide access to performance data, and encourage innovation, learning will happen organically. They invest in workshops, dashboards, and communication platforms. They celebrate improvement projects and share success stories.

Three years later, they discover that learning remains isolated and episodic. Some teams improve some things sometimes. But there's no systematic capability to identify problems, test solutions, measure results, and spread what works. Learning happens by accident, not by design.

The problem isn't a lack of tools or training. The problem is the absence of three foundational capabilities that enable everything else. Without these three, your improvement methods don't get used, your data doesn't drive decisions, and your innovations don't spread. With these three, transformation accelerates because the organization has infrastructure for continuous learning.

Let me be clear about what I mean by "capability." I'm not talking about knowledge or skills that individuals possess. I'm talking about organizational infrastructure that enables collective action regardless of who is present. When key people leave—and they will—capability persists because it's embedded in systems, processes, and culture rather than dependent on particular personalities.

The three essential capabilities are psychological safety, quality improvement mentoring, and data-driven learning cycles. These aren't optional enhancements. They're foundational infrastructure. Without all three, learning organization development fails. With all three, it succeeds.

Let me show you what each capability is, why it matters, and how to build it.

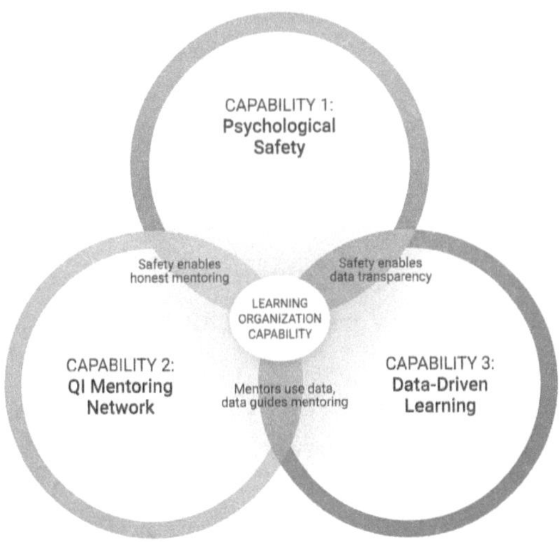

. . .

CAPABILITY ONE: PSYCHOLOGICAL SAFETY

Psychological safety is the shared confidence that interpersonal risks—such as raising concerns, admitting errors, seeking help, and challenging assumptions—are safe to take without fear of shame, rejection, or punishment. Organizations with high psychological safety continuously learn because members bring issues to light early, try new approaches without fear of failure, and openly share knowledge. Conversely, organizations with low psychological safety may seem functional yet fragile—problems remain hidden until they become crises, people conceal mistakes rather than learn from them, and innovation stalls because no one dares to suggest new ideas.

Amy Edmondson's research shows that psychological safety is a key predictor of organizational learning and performance. Interestingly, she found a paradox: high-performing teams with strong psychological safety tend to report higher error rates than lower-performing teams. This doesn't imply they make more mistakes; instead, they are more likely to report them. In contrast, low-performing teams lacking psychological safety tend to hide errors, which hampers learning and allows problems to grow.

I observed this pattern at an academic medical center that was working to reduce hospital-acquired infections. They launched a vigorous campaign urging frontline staff to report near-misses and process failures, set up online reporting systems, and promoted a blame-free culture. After six months, they had collected many reports, but only from specific units. The ICU reported dozens of near-misses each month, while the surgical units reported almost none.

The chief nursing officer was confused. "Are our surgical units really that much better at preventing infections?" she inquired. No, they weren't. During confidential interviews with surgical nurses, they recounted similar process failures in their units. However, they didn't report these issues because, in the past, when they voiced concerns about physician conduct or procedural breaches, they faced retaliation. This wasn't formal punishment but more subtle forms—hostile glances, social exclusion, physicians becoming "too busy" to respond to questions. Junior nurses learned to stay silent.

Meanwhile, the ICU fostered real psychological safety because its leadership actively supported open dissent. When nurses voiced concerns about procedures, physicians responded with public thanks. Reports of near-misses prompted curiosity about root causes instead of blame. As a result, ICU nurses felt comfortable speaking up and did so. Conversely, surgical nurses felt unsafe and remained silent.

Building psychological safety isn't focused on communication campaigns or values statements. Instead, it's about how leaders react to bad news, mistakes, and differing opinions. It is shaped by specific moments—the time a concern is raised about a senior physician's conduct, when a junior resident admits to missing a diagnosis, or when a frontline nurse recommends an improved workflow.

When leaders respond with curiosity, gratitude, and a focus on solving problems, psychological safety strengthens. Conversely, if they react defensively, blame others, or punish—even subtly through tone or body language—psychological safety diminishes. Once lost, it can take years to restore, as people tend to remember being punished for honesty much more than being rewarded for it.

Building psychological safety involves consistent leadership behavior change rather than mere words. Leaders should demonstrate vulnerability by publicly acknowledging their mistakes. They need to handle inquiries rather than reach immediate conclusions. When receiving bad news, they should first express appreciation—"thank you for bringing this forward"—before asking, "what happened?" Leaders must establish explicit meeting norms, such as "we expect everyone to contribute" and "disagreement fosters better thinking," and ensure these norms are upheld by guiding discussions when louder voices drown out quieter ones.

They must also confront toxic behaviors that undermine psychological safety, such as the brilliant surgeon who berates residents, the department chair punishing dissent, and the senior nurse fostering hostility toward newer staff. Leaders often overlook these actions because the individuals involved are high performers or politically influential. However, allowing toxic behavior to persist day to day communicates a simple message: performance is more important than safety. When this message is received, psychological safety can no longer thrive.

Measuring psychological safety goes beyond using engagement surveys with generic questions. It requires observing specific behaviors, such as whether people speak up in meetings or defer to hierarchy. When errors occur, are they openly discussed or concealed? Do junior staff share ideas proactively or wait for instructions? Do team members challenge senior leaders, or do they tell them what they want to hear? These behaviors should be tracked systematically through observation and confidential interviews, rather than relying solely on survey scores that can be manipulated.

Building psychological safety requires eighteen to thirty-six months of consistent leadership actions. It cannot be hastened through workshops or posters. Instead, it develops through countless small interactions in which leaders respond to vulnerability with respect rather than punishment. Once established, psychological safety becomes self-sustaining. This leads to increased speaking up, earlier problem resolution, more innovations, and an organization that truly learns from experience.

Psychological safety is essential for effective transformation. Without it, people are unlikely to adopt new methods, share data, or suggest changes due to fear of failure or criticism. It serves as the crucial foundation that supports all other capabilities.

THE UNCOMFORTABLE TRUTH

You can't build psychological safety while protecting toxic high-performers. Every time someone misbehaves and faces no consequences, everyone else learns that safety only applies to some people. If you're unwilling to address the surgeon everyone is afraid of, stop pretending you're building a learning organization.

THE DECISION POINT

A nurse reports to you that Dr. Chen—a beloved physician, major research grant holder, and 30-year veteran—berated a resident in front of a patient's family for questioning his medication order. The resident was correct; the order contained an error that Dr. Chen refused to acknowledge.

This is the third such report about Dr. Chen this year. Previous concerns were "addressed" through informal conversations that changed nothing.

Dr. Chen generates $2M in research grants and is considered irreplaceable in his specialty. He has powerful allies on the medical staff. He is also systematically destroying psychological safety in every clinical area he touches.

You have publicly committed to building psychological safety.

What do you do?

Be specific. Don't say "address the behavior"—say exactly what you would do, when you would do it, and what happens if Dr. Chen refuses to change.

If your answer involves "coaching," "mentoring," or "counseling" without clear consequences for continued behavior, you're not building psychological safety. You're protecting a toxic high-performer while pretending to care about culture.

If your answer involves immediate escalation to formal consequences, ask yourself: Are you actually willing to lose $2M in research grants and a specialty leader over "interpersonal issues"? Will your board support you?

The residents and nurses in your organization already know how you'll answer this question. They've seen how you handle Dr. Chen and people like him for years. What you do—not what you say—defines your actual commitment to psychological safety.

What I would actually do: ______________________________

____

CAPABILITY TWO: QUALITY IMPROVEMENT MENTORING

Most organizations treat quality improvement training as if it were academic education. They send staff to workshops, teach PDSA or Lean tools, and sometimes certify them in Six Sigma, expecting them to lead improvements upon return. This approach sometimes succeeds—especially with motivated individuals in supportive settings—but often fails because knowing the methods doesn't ensure effective application in complex organizational environments.

Mastering improvement leadership is more like learning surgery than studying anatomy. While textbooks provide knowledge of anatomy, hands-on practice under experienced supervision is essential to learn surgery. Likewise, understanding PDSA cycles in a classroom isn't enough to lead to actual organizational change; mentoring from someone with proven success is crucial.

This is why the second crucial capability is a mentorship network for quality improvement—comprising experienced improvement leaders who mentor frontline teams on real projects, sharing knowledge through hands-on apprenticeships rather than traditional classroom training.

The hub-and-spoke model discussed in Chapter 2 was successful in part because Riverside Health System invested significantly in training QI mentors. They chose twenty-five individuals based on their clinical credibility, focus on improvement, and coaching skills.

These mentors received comprehensive training in various improvement methods, including PDSA, Lean, measurement techniques, change management, and facilitation. Crucially, they also established a community of practice in which mentors could share experiences and learn from one another's challenges.

The twenty-five mentors collaborated directly with spoke teams on real improvement projects. They did not just facilitate workshops; they were on-site, observing workflows, asking questions, assisting teams in framing problems, guiding them through change cycles, troubleshooting barriers, interpreting data, and gradually transferring skills so teams could operate independently.

This apprenticeship model is effective because it bridges the gap between understanding methods and applying them. A frontline team may grasp the PDSA cycle conceptually but find it challenging to formulate a change hypothesis tailored to their workflow. They might be aware of the importance of measuring results, but are unsure about which metrics to track. While they comprehend stakeholder engagement in theory, they could freeze when faced with resistance from the department chair. Mentors play a crucial role in guiding teams through these real-world challenges that no workshop can predict.

Successful QI mentoring depends on choosing suitable individuals and nurturing their development. Effective mentors are trusted by clinical staff because they understand real clinical practice, not just theoretical concepts. They possess improvement skills acquired by leading numerous successful initiatives, not merely through training attendance. Additionally, they demonstrate coaching abilities—they guide without micromanaging, ask insightful questions rather than give direct solutions, and gradually transfer skills to foster independence.

Building effective mentors demands a significant commitment of time and resources. Allocate at least forty hours for comprehensive training on improvement methods, change management, coaching, and adult learning principles. Support continuous growth through monthly community-of-practice meetings where mentors share experiences and tackle challenges collectively. Ensure mentors have dedicated time for mentoring activities, as they cannot adequately support improvement initiatives if these tasks are left to their limited free time after regular duties.

Most importantly, develop career pathways that make QI mentoring appealing to talented individuals. Suppose mentoring remains volunteer work without recognition or advancement opportunities. In that case, you'll only attract those with free time, not your top talent. Effective organizations establish formal positions such as QI director, improvement coach, or clinical transformation specialist, offering proper compensation, authority, and clear career growth. They also incorporate improvement leadership into promotion criteria and publicly celebrate mentors.

The mentor-to-team ratio is essential. Typically, one mentor can effectively oversee three to five improvement projects simultaneously. When projects exceed five, the quality of support declines because mentors become overstretched. Therefore, if you have 20 improvement projects, you'll need about 4 to 7 active mentors. It's better to plan for sufficient mentoring capacity rather than assuming just a few people can handle unlimited projects.

Monitor mentor effectiveness systematically. Do the teams they mentor complete their projects successfully? Do those teams develop the ability to lead future projects independently? Do the projects produce and maintain measurable improvements? These outcome metrics show whether your mentoring truly builds capability or merely fosters dependency.

Developing a mentoring network typically takes twelve to eighteen months, from selecting mentors to completing initial projects. This process can't be hurried, as mentors require time to gain expertise, and teams need time to build their capabilities with guidance. Once the network is established, it becomes self-sustaining and scalable. Experienced mentors train new mentors, and successful teams often mentor newer ones, creating a compounding effect on capabilities.

Without a mentoring network, your improvement efforts rely on a limited number of experts. When these individuals leave or become overwhelmed, progress stalls. Establishing a strong mentoring network enables the spread of improvement skills across the organization, ensuring continuity even when personnel change and allowing growth beyond initial initiatives.

THE UNCOMFORTABLE TRUTH

Training people in QI methods is easy. Getting them to actually use those methods—consistently, over time, even when it's inconvenient—is hard. Most organizations have trained far more people in PDSA than are actually doing PDSA. Certificates of completion are not evidence of capability.

CAPABILITY THREE: DATA-DRIVEN LEARNING CYCLES

The third crucial capability is the systematic use of data to foster learning and guide decisions. This isn't about data for reporting, compliance, or just defending existing decisions—it's about using data for learning purposes. It includes data that highlights when processes fail, shows whether implemented changes have actually improved results, detects unwarranted variations needing correction, and supports quick testing and refinement.

Most academic health systems are overwhelmed with data but lack genuine insights. They utilize advanced electronic health records that record millions of data points and generate numerous reports. They monitor hundreds of metrics. However, when leaders are asked if their sepsis protocol lowers mortality, they often cannot provide a confident answer. Similarly, when asked whether a recent workflow change has enhanced efficiency, they tend to shrug. Despite this abundance of data, they suffer from a scarcity of meaningful learning.

The core issue isn't the lack of data, but rather the absence of structured processes that connect data to decision-making. While data exists in various systems, it doesn't reach the right people at the right time in usable formats. By the time data is extracted, cleaned, analyzed, and reported, weeks or months may have passed, eliminating the chance for quick learning. Additionally, even if data arrives promptly, many struggle to interpret it correctly—they can't distinguish real signals from random noise, aren't sure how to test if observed changes truly caused improvements, and lack frameworks to turn data into practical insights.

Developing data-driven learning abilities depends on three key elements: available data infrastructure, analytical skills, and structured review processes.

Accessible data infrastructure enables you to retrieve essential data within hours or days rather than weeks or months. It involves robust data warehouses that consolidate data from various systems, analytics tools that enable fast querying and visualization, and direct team access to track their metrics without relying on central analysts. Building this infrastructure requires substantial investment in technology, data governance, and analytics expertise. However, without it, learning stays theoretical because measuring actual improvements becomes impossible.

Analytic capability involves understanding how to use data for learning rather than just reporting. This entails training in statistical process control to differentiate signals from noise, interpreting run charts to spot trends and shifts, and measurement for improvement to develop suitable metrics and data collection methods. Don't assume that clinical training alone has prepared people for this—while physicians and nurses are excellent clinicians, many lack sufficient statistical literacy. Offer practical analytics training focused on improvement rather than purely academic statistics courses.

Systematic review processes establish a regular schedule for analyzing data and implementing insights. This involves daily huddles where teams assess the previous day's performance and highlight issues requiring urgent action; weekly meetings to review metrics and discuss obstacles; monthly departmental evaluations to monitor progress toward goals and refine strategies; and quarterly system-wide reviews to identify trends across units and allocate resources accordingly.

The main point is "systematic." These reviews occur regularly, regardless of whether anyone feels like it. They follow standard agendas to ensure data is thoroughly examined. The process yields documented decisions with clear accountability. This shifts data review from an optional activity dependent on memory to a mandated process integrated into operations.

I observed this capability develop within a health system that initially faced challenges with data-driven learning. Although they had robust data systems, they lacked systematic review processes. The data was available, but did not influence decision-making. Their solution was straightforward: each clinical unit started a fifteen-minute daily huddle to review the previous day's key metrics—such as patient flow, safety incidents, satisfaction scores, and staff concerns. They displayed run charts illustrating trends over time. When metrics indicated issues, the huddles prompted immediate actions and straightforward assignment of responsibilities.

Within six months, the daily huddles profoundly transformed the organization's operations. Issues were identified and resolved within hours rather than weeks. Process improvements occurred quickly as teams observed immediate results in their metrics. Staff engagement grew because employees recognized that measurement prompted action, not just reporting that went unnoticed.

Creating data-driven learning cycles typically takes six to twelve months, depending on the initial infrastructure. Starting from scratch usually takes more time, while those with existing systems that need cultural shifts around data use can establish new norms within six months through systematic implementation.

Without data-driven learning cycles, progress relies on opinions. People debate the effectiveness of changes, relying on anecdotes and impressions rather than evidence. Implementing strong data cycles accelerates learning by enabling quick identification of what works and what doesn't, facilitating faster improvement.

THE UNCOMFORTABLE TRUTH

Most healthcare "data" isn't information—it's noise. Dashboards full of metrics that no one acts on aren't learning tools; they're performance theater. If you can't name three decisions that were made differently because of data in the past month, your data systems are decorative, not functional.

HOW THE THREE CAPABILITIES INTERCONNECT

These three capabilities are interconnected and mutually supportive. Psychological safety allows teams to discuss data that may reveal uncomfortable truths openly. QI mentoring helps teams understand data and develop better measurement methods. Data-driven learning provides evidence of progress, boosting confidence and encouraging ongoing effort.

When all three elements are present, a virtuous cycle occurs: teams leverage data to find problems, openly discuss root causes, and receive mentoring to test solutions. Data then indicates whether the changes are effective, boosting learning and building capability. Over time, this process enhances the organization's ability to improve continuously.

When any one is absent, the cycle is disrupted. Without psychological safety, data tends to be concealed or distorted. Without mentoring, teams struggle to turn data into actionable insights. Without data cycles, learning stays anecdotal and lacks validation.

This is why these three are essential and cannot be compromised. You can't make up for poor psychological safety with improved data systems. Training workshops can't replace genuine mentoring. Occasional dashboards aren't a substitute for systematic data review. All three are necessary for a learning organization to operate effectively.

The timeline for completing all three runs spans eighteen to thirty-six months from start to finish. While you can speed up the process by running efforts in parallel, the essential work for each cannot be shortened. Recognize that capability building requires time, invest suitably, and track progress consistently.

By month eighteen, you should see tangible improvements in psychological safety, a functioning mentor network supporting various projects, and systematic data review processes integrated into daily operations. By month thirty-six, these capabilities are expected to become self-sustaining—with psychological safety upheld through consistent leadership practices, mentors training new mentors, and data review cycles becoming routine rather than requiring enforcement.

At this stage, you've established real learning organization capability. It's not just about attending workshops or setting up governance structures; you've built the infrastructure that supports large-scale, ongoing learning.

Now, I'll highlight the common mistakes that can undermine these capabilities even after they've been developed. Knowing what to build isn't enough—you also need to understand how to preserve and not destroy what you've created.

Why All Three Are Non-Negotiable

WITHOUT Psychological Safety:

→ People hide mistakes instead of learning from them
→ Data gets manipulated to look good, not reveal truth
→ Mentoring becomes performance theater, not development

WITHOUT QI Mentoring Network:

→ Training doesn't translate to actual improvement capability
→ Teams struggle without expert guidance on real problems
→ Improvement efforts remain dependent on few individuals

WITHOUT Data-Driven Learning Cycles:

→ Can't verify if improvements actually worked
→ Decisions based on opinion/anecdote, not evidence
→ Unable to distinguish real improvement from noise

⚠ You cannot skip one and compensate with the other two.
All three must exist for learning organization capability to function.

BEFORE YOU CONTINUE

The three capabilities—psychological safety, QI mentoring, and data-driven learning—are interdependent. Weakness in one undermines the others. Assess honestly where you stand.

1. Name the highest-revenue physician in your organization who has demonstrated unprofessional behavior in the past year. What happened to them? If the answer is "nothing meaningful," your psychological safety initiative is performative. People know who is protected and who isn't.

2. How many staff in your organization have been formally trained in quality improvement methodology? Not "attended a workshop"—actually trained with ongoing coaching and project completion? If the number is below 1% of your workforce, you don't have QI capability; you have QI awareness.

Number of trained QI practitioners: _______

Total workforce: _______

Percentage: _______%

3. If you wanted to know your current sepsis mortality rate right now—not tomorrow, not next week, but right now—could you get that number? How long would it take? If the answer is more than a few hours, your data infrastructure cannot support learning organization development.

4. Think of a time in the past year when your organization learned something from a failure—not just investigated it, but actually changed practice as a result. How long did that change take to implement across relevant areas? If you can't think of an example, or if it took more than three months, your learning cycle is too slow.

5. Of the three capabilities, which is your organization's weakest? Be specific about why. This is where you should focus first—but be warned that leaders often overestimate their psychological safety because they don't hear the truth, they've made it unsafe to speak.

Weakest capability: ______________________________

Why: ____

6

COMMON PITFALLS AND HOW TO AVOID THEM

SIX WAYS ORGANIZATIONS DESTROY TRANSFORMATION EVEN AFTER INITIAL SUCCESS

THE MOMENT OF VULNERABILITY

You've handled everything correctly. You've set up clear governance and used your initial 90 days to lay a solid foundation, rather than rushing into implementation. You're steadily working on three key capabilities—psychological safety, QI mentoring, and data-driven learning cycles. The early outcomes look promising. Stakeholders are involved, and the board supports your efforts. You're moving forward as planned.

This is the point of greatest vulnerability.

It's not that you're failing; it's that you're succeeding. Successful moments can lead to complacency, overconfidence, and the gradual weakening of the disciplines that initially brought you success.

I've observed more transformations stumble during periods of apparent success than during periods of obvious failure. When problems are evident, leaders tend to focus and adjust their course. However, when things seem to be going smoothly, they lower their guard. They assume the transformation is self-sustaining, shifting focus to other priorities. Small compromises, which seem reasonable at the time, can accumulate and lead to the collapse of the transformation.

Let me highlight the six most common ways organizations undermine successful transformations. These aren't just theoretical risks; they are patterns I've seen repeatedly in institutions that worked hard to build capability, made genuine progress, and then unintentionally reversed it through predictable mistakes.

The good news is that all six issues can be entirely avoided if you identify them early and stay disciplined. However, the bad news is that simply recognizing them isn't enough—you need to consciously resist these patterns, especially when everything seems fine.

PITFALL ONE: DECLARING VICTORY TOO EARLY

Eighteen months into your transformation, your metrics are impressive. Hospital-acquired infections decreased by 25%. Readmissions are down 15%. Staff engagement scores have increased by 18 points. Patient satisfaction ranks in the 90th percentile. The improvement projects you've launched are delivering results. People are speaking the language of continuous improvement. Quick wins have become sustained gains.

The board wants to celebrate your achievements. The CEO grants interviews to healthcare publications that highlight your transformational success, while internal communications emphasize your accomplishments. You're invited to speak at national conferences, and other health systems are eager to learn from your experience.

This is precisely when most transformations start to fade.

The issue isn't celebrating progress itself—acknowledging achievements helps sustain momentum and morale. The real challenge is the subtle transition from thinking, "we're making progress and need to keep pushing," to "we've achieved our goal and can shift focus." This shift begins subtly: the steering committee that used to meet monthly now meets quarterly, resources once dedicated to capability building are redirected elsewhere, and other demands gradually take over protected time for improvement. Attention begins to drift away.

I observed this at a West Coast academic medical center that achieved impressive results in its first two years. They genuinely cultivated psychological safety, developed a strong mentor network, and set up efficient data cycles. Their clinical outcomes significantly advanced, and leadership rightly took pride in their achievements.

Then they announced the completion of the transformation. The steering committee, which had overseen governance and accountability, was disbanded. The chief learning officer was reassigned to different duties. They ceased training new QI mentors, citing "we have enough." Meanwhile, they shifted improvement resources toward a new strategic goal—expanding population health.

Within a year, their progress started to decline. Psychological safety declined as new leaders, unfamiliar with learning organization principles, made traditional decisions. The mentor network shrank as mentors became overwhelmed without continuous support and training. Data review sessions grew infrequent and ultimately halted. Improvement initiatives that had been maintained no longer yielded results.

By year four, they nearly reverted to their original state. This wasn't due to flawed initial efforts but rather to their ceasing to practice it before it became deeply integrated into the organization's core practices.

Here's the reality: Transformation is an ongoing process. Learning organizations don't simply "become" learning organizations and automatically maintain that state. They stay that way by practicing consistent discipline and continually renewing capabilities. Once you see the transformation as complete, that's when it starts to fall apart.

How can you avoid this trap? Establish transformation infrastructure as a permanent part of the organization instead of a temporary project. Your governance structures—such as the steering committee or the System Learning Council—should operate indefinitely. The chief learning officer, or a similar role, should be a permanent position, not a temporary one. QI mentor training should continue in cohorts to keep capabilities current as roles and personnel change. Data review cycles should become routine procedures rather than special projects. Improvement efforts need to be integrated into job descriptions and performance metrics, rather than viewed as voluntary extra duties.

When you achieve early wins, share them as proof that your approach is effective, not as an indicator that the work is finished. "This progress demonstrates that our capabilities are growing. To maintain and extend these gains, ongoing investment and discipline are necessary." Present success as a reason to reinforce what is working, rather than an excuse to shift resources elsewhere.

THE UNCOMFORTABLE TRUTH

The initiative you declared a success last year probably isn't. Look at the metrics now, not the metrics from the launch celebration. If you don't know the current numbers, that's your answer. Most "successful" transformation initiatives are just initiatives that leadership stopped paying attention to after the initial results came in.

THE DECISION POINT

It's month 18 of your transformation. Early results are strong: three quick wins achieved, governance structures functioning, 15 QI mentors trained, and staff engagement scores improving. Your board is pleased. Your CEO has asked you to present "transformation success" at the next all-hands meeting.

You know the reality is more complicated. The quick wins were in receptive departments. Two of your most challenging departments haven't engaged at all. Your governance council hasn't yet faced a severe test of its authority. You're not sure whether staff engagement improvements will sustain or if they only reflect temporary optimism.

The CEO wants a victory narrative. The board wants validation that their investment is paying off. Frontline staff want to believe transformation is real this time.

What do you present?

If you present the victory narrative the CEO wants, you risk creating the very premature victory declaration this chapter warns against. When the more complex work of years 2-3 begins, the organization will expect smooth sailing—and be demoralized when it doesn't come.

If you present a more honest "progress with significant challenges ahead" message, you risk disappointing leadership and undermining the momentum you've built. Organizational attention is finite, and pessimism can become self-fulfilling.

How do you honor the real progress while preventing the complacency that premature victory creates? What exactly would you say?

The key message I would deliver: ______________________

____

____

PITFALL TWO: TOLERATING TOXIC HIGH PERFORMERS

You're systematically fostering psychological safety. Leaders demonstrate vulnerability, react to bad news with curiosity, and promote diverse viewpoints. Teams increasingly share their thoughts more openly. You can observe a cultural change taking place.

Then, your leading cardiac surgeon—earning $15 million annually—berates a resident in front of the entire surgical team. Alternatively, your department chair, who secures $20 million in research funding, dismisses a nurse raising a patient safety concern. Additionally, the highest-billing hospitalist group refuses to adopt the new sepsis protocol, claiming, "We know better than the protocol developers."

This moment determines whether psychological safety is genuine or merely superficial. By confronting the behavior head-on and making it clear that strong clinical or financial results do not excuse actions that harm psychological safety, you reinforce the culture. Conversely, accepting such behavior because of the individual's income or influence immediately and completely damages psychological safety.

Everyone in your organization is paying attention right now. If high performers display toxic behavior and it is ignored, it sends a strong message: while we claim to value psychological safety, performance, and authority take precedence. This creates a perception that psychological safety is not genuine. Observers who see toxic acts being tolerated will be hesitant to speak out in the future. They will realize that the official values do not truly influence organizational behavior.

I've observed institutions investing millions in culture-change efforts and extensively training leaders in psychological safety. They often make genuine progress, but then undo it all by neglecting to address a single high-revenue toxic individual. The impact goes beyond the initial incident, as it sets a precedent for similar behavior to be tolerated. It also signals that organizational values can be compromised depending on an individual's economic importance.

This trap is especially subtle because leaders justify their actions as pragmatic. They might say, "We can't afford to lose Dr. Johnson, who would oversee the cardiac surgery program?" or "Professor Smith secures too much research funding," or "This hospitalist group brings in essential revenue." Such reasoning overlooks the actual costs of tolerance: excellent individuals leaving because they won't endure toxic environments, difficulty attracting talented clinicians with options, ongoing psychological harm to staff, and the erosion of the organization's ability to change.

How can you prevent this pitfall? Set explicit behavioral standards that are non-negotiable for all staff, regardless of their performance or role. When toxic behavior appears, handle it promptly and straightforwardly. Have a private talk and clearly state that the behavior is unacceptable and needs to change. If it persists, enforce progressive consequences, including termination if required.

Some top performers will alter their behavior when faced with real consequences, while others will choose to leave. Allow them to go. Losing a revenue-generating team member causes short-term disruption, but it is much less costly than permitting behavior that harms the organizational culture. Often, once toxic high performers depart, team performance actually improves as people no longer operate in fear.

Communicate these decisions and their reasoning openly. When staff observe that behavioral standards are enforced even for influential individuals, psychological safety significantly improves. This shows that the organization's values are genuine, not just aspirational.

PITFALL THREE: GOVERNANCE EROSION

You established clear governance by selecting a model—centralized, federated, or hub-and-spoke—that the board approved, with explicit authority and accountability. You then implemented it, and it is now functioning effectively.

Gradually and subtly, governance diminishes. The System Learning Council, which previously had budget authority, finds its decisions increasingly reviewed by executives before they are enacted. The power to require protocol adoption becomes no more than a suggestion to "strongly encourage" compliance. Department chairs opposing system initiatives realize they can ignore them without repercussions. Matters that governance frameworks are meant to decide are often escalated to executives who were not intended to be part of the decision process.

This erosion seldom occurs through direct reversal. No one states "we're abandoning hub-and-spoke governance." Instead, it evolves through countless small compromises. For example, a department chair strongly objects to a system protocol, but instead of enforcing it, you grant a one-time exception. A hospital president persuades the CEO that they require special treatment due to their unique situation. The System Learning Council suggests discontinuing a poorly performing initiative, but executives override this decision because of the significant investments already made.

Each compromise may seem reasonable on its own, and each exception looks justified by specific circumstances. However, taken together, they suggest that governance isn't truly firm—decisions can be appealed, mandates are just suggestions, and authority is negotiable.

I observed governance decline at a Midwest academic health system that had effectively adopted a hub-and-spoke model with real authority. Their System Learning Council demonstrated its value by making sound decisions, ensuring accountability, and delivering measurable progress. However, when a new hospital president from outside the system arrived, he viewed the governance structure as restrictive and campaigned to the CEO for greater independence. In an effort to keep the new leader, the CEO allowed deviations from standard governance rules.

Other site leaders observed this and called for similar autonomy. Within six months, hub-and-spoke governance became merely symbolic, with each site functioning independently and the System Learning Council relegated to an advisory role. The ongoing transformation slowed, and progress on improvements halted. The organization began to fragment again, undoing the governance structure it had aimed to establish.

How can you prevent this mistake? Consider governance authority as absolute. When your governance bodies make decisions within their set powers, those decisions are final. There are no appeals to higher authorities, no special privileges for influential individuals, and no case-by-case negotiations.

This calls for discipline from the board and executives. When an appeal regarding governance is made to you, your reply should be: "That decision falls under the System Learning Council's authority. I support their judgment. If you think they erred, discuss it with them directly, not with me." By directing appeals to the proper governance body, you reaffirm that their authority is legitimate.

Also, establish clear processes for evolving governance. Governance models should adapt over time in response to new insights and changing conditions. However, any adaptation should occur through intentional governance review and updates, not through informal decline. Plan annual governance reviews to assess the effectiveness of current structures, implement explicit changes if necessary, and reaffirm your commitment to the existing governance framework.

> THE UNCOMFORTABLE TRUTH
>
> *Governance doesn't fail dramatically; it erodes slowly. Each small exception, each "one-time" accommodation, each decision to avoid conflict weakens the structure. By the time you notice governance has decayed, you've lost the authority to restore it without a major confrontation you've been trying to avoid.*

PITFALL FOUR: UNDER-INVESTING IN CAPABILITY RENEWAL

You invested significantly in developing initial capabilities by training 25 QI mentors, building a strong data infrastructure, and establishing systematic review processes. The skills and systems you've put in place are functioning effectively and yielding positive results.

Then, you cease investing in capability renewal. You don't initiate training for new mentor cohorts because you believe "we have enough mentors already." You postpone technology upgrades, reasoning that "the current system works fine." You cut training budgets, assuming "people already know the methods." You assume that once capability is developed, it sustains itself.

Capability diminishes over time due to natural attrition and obsolescence. People leave—retiring, being promoted, or moving to different roles. Technology also ages, becoming outdated, while methods change, rendering initial training inadequate. Without ongoing capability renewal, what has been built gradually degrades and eventually ceases to function.

I observed an East Coast system that had developed a strong mentor network of 30 individuals. Five years later, half of them had transitioned to different roles or left the organization. The remaining mentors were overwhelmed, trying to support the same number of projects with only half the staff. They ceased developing new mentors because training seemed like a luxury when they were already stretched thin. As a result, the mentor network collapsed under the load, eliminating the group's capacity for improvement.

How can you prevent this mistake? Integrate continuous capability renewal into your operating model. Annually train new QI mentor cohorts, regardless of immediate needs, to develop a steady pipeline of expertise as staff shift roles. Allocate budget for regular technology updates and upgrades. Offer ongoing education to mentors to keep their skills up to date. Consider capability investment as a continual operational expense rather than a one-time capital expenditure.

Also, establish redundancy in key capabilities to avoid single points of failure that could be compromised if one person leaves. Distribute expertise among multiple individuals and document processes to ensure knowledge isn't confined to just some people. While this redundancy incurs additional costs, it safeguards against catastrophic capability loss when key personnel depart.

PITFALL FIVE: SCALING BEFORE YOU'RE READY

Your pilot projects have yielded excellent results, demonstrating that the hub is operating effectively. Early adopter spoke sites are successfully implementing the system. You are now eager to accelerate progress and involve all remaining sites.

This eagerness can result in premature scaling, such as engaging twenty spoke sites at once when capacity is only five. It causes the launch of system-wide initiatives before testing and refining approaches on a smaller scale. Additionally, successful interventions in specific contexts are often implemented in other settings without adequate adaptation, risking ineffectiveness.

Premature scaling overstresses your mentoring capacity. Mentors who effectively managed three projects at once become less effective when supporting ten. This leads to a decline in implementation quality. Teams do not get enough support. Projects often fail not because of flawed interventions but because of poor implementation.

How can you prevent this mistake? Approach scaling systematically by considering real capacity rather than idealistic deadlines. Use the mentor-to-project ratio—one mentor supporting three to five projects simultaneously—to decide how many sites to involve. With 10 mentors, aim to work on no more than 30 to 50 projects. Hold off on training more mentors until you're ready to handle additional sites.

Also, establish clear criteria for scaling readiness. Sites should meet specific minimum standards before engagement, including confirmed leadership commitment, operational data systems, identified local champions, and allocated resources. Do not engage sites with the expectation that they will develop their readiness during implementation. Ensure readiness is demonstrated before starting.

PITFALL SIX: MEASUREMENT THEATER

You set up metrics to monitor transformation progress and created dashboards to display performance data. You review these metrics regularly. However, over time, they often become more about appearances than useful learning tools.

Teams often present game metrics that suggest improvement, even when no real progress was made. Leaders tend to celebrate reaching targets without considering if those achievements create real value. Dashboard reviews turn into performance displays rather than authentic learning discussions. The focus shifts from asking, "What are we learning and how do we improve?" to making the numbers look better.

This occurs when penalties for poor metrics are punitive instead of supportive. When missing targets leads to blame rather than encouraging problem-solving, individuals tend to manipulate metrics rather than genuinely improve performance. Similarly, when achieving targets leads to rewards regardless of the actual benefit to patients, the focus shifts to optimizing metrics rather than achieving meaningful outcomes.

To avoid this pitfall, differentiate between learning and accountability metrics. Use learning metrics to guide improvement efforts without penalizing unfavorable trends. Save accountability metrics for well-established processes where there is clear evidence connecting metric performance to patient outcomes.

Also, regularly perform data quality audits to ensure that the metrics accurately reflect reality. When teams demonstrate significant improvement, confirm these results via direct observation and additional data sources. If metrics improve but staff report no changes in their workflows, investigate whether the improvement is genuine or just a measurement artifact.

THE UNCOMFORTABLE TRUTH

If your frontline staff are cynical about your dashboards, the dashboards are the problem, not the staff. Metrics that can be gamed will be gamed. Metrics that don't drive decisions are ignored. Metrics that punish honesty destroy the data you need to actually improve. Ask yourself: do people trust your measurement system, or do they work around it?

MAINTAINING DISCIPLINE

These six pitfalls follow a similar pattern: they are easier to succumb to than to prevent. Declaring victory too soon often seems tempting after significant achievements. Tolerating toxic high performers can seem necessary when they bring in revenue. Permitting governance deterioration might appear like practical flexibility. Under-investing in capability renewal seems like saving resources. Premature scaling can seem like striving for growth. Measurement theater disguises superficial accountability.

Avoiding these pitfalls demands ongoing discipline, particularly when everything appears to be fine. It involves making decisions that may seem overly cautious or strict, and maintaining structures and investments that might seem unnecessary.

This discipline may seem dull because it doesn't produce conference presentations or publications. However, it's essential work that involves maintaining what you've built so it can develop into real organizational capability.

This discipline is what differentiates successful transformations from those that only show early promise and then fail. Focus on doing the hard work of developing capability, and then dedicate equal effort to protecting and maintaining what you've achieved.

The ultimate success of your transformation hinges less on your initial steps and more on your ability to stay disciplined over the years until learning organization capability is fully integrated into the company's core DNA.

That's what the conclusion is about: What happens next, now that you know what to do and what to avoid.

BEFORE YOU CONTINUE

These six pitfalls don't announce themselves. They feel like success until they become a failure. Be honest about which ones you're most vulnerable to.

1. When was the last time your organization declared victory on a transformation initiative? What metrics did you use? Look at those metrics now—not the launch metrics, the current metrics. If you don't know the current numbers, that's your answer about whether the victory was premature.

2. Name the highest-performing individual in your organization whose behavior undermines psychological safety. You know who this is. Everyone knows. What would have to change for you to address their behavior? If your answer involves waiting for them to retire, you've chosen what kind of organization you're building.

3. Look at your governance structures from 18 months ago. Are they stronger now, weaker, or about the same? Governance decay happens slowly and invisibly. If you haven't actively reinforced your governance authority in the past six months, it has probably weakened.

4. How much of your improvement capability is concentrated in a small number of people? If your top three QI mentors left tomorrow, what would happen? Sustainable capability is distributed capability. If you're dependent on a few individuals, you're vulnerable.

5. Think about your measurement systems. Do you measure what actually matters, or do you measure what's easy to measure? Are your metrics driving behavior, or are they being gamed? If you're not sure, ask frontline staff what they think of your dashboards. Their cynicism will tell you everything.

6. Of the six pitfalls in this chapter, which one are you most likely to fall into, given your organization's culture and your own tendencies? Please write it down. Now write down what you will do differently to avoid it.

MOST LIKELY PITFALL: ______________________________

WHAT I WILL DO DIFFERENTLY: __________________________

PART III

CONCLUSION

YOUR TRANSFORMATION STARTS NOW

THE CHOICE YOU FACE AND YOUR FIRST THREE ACTIONS

THE CALL YOU MAKE

Recall the late-night call that started this book? The CEO was shattered by yet another avoidable death, confused as to why her top-tier academic medical center continued to struggle with basic infection control, despite having protocols, training, and dashboards in place.

Imagine a different call with the same CEO, eighteen months later, but with a completely different tone.

She says, "I need to tell you what happened today," but this time her voice is energetic rather than exhausted. "We have now gone six months without a central line infection in our ICU," she announces. 'Six months, after years of this being our ongoing issue.' She adds that the protocol has been adopted across all units, not just the ICU. Surgical teams have been asked to adapt it to their workflows, and the emergency department is testing a version for peripheral lines.

She pauses and says, "But what truly matters is this. During our daily huddle this morning, a first-year resident voiced a concern about hand hygiene compliance in a specific area. Two years ago, she wouldn't have spoken up—too inexperienced and risky. Now, the attending physician publicly thanked her and quickly assembled a team to fix the issue. That moment made me realize that something essential has shifted. We're not only preventing infections but also evolving into a learning organization."

This is achievable, not just aspirational. It happens when you genuinely develop the capability of a learning organization.

WHAT YOU NOW KNOW

You've gone through six chapters that reveal insights about transformation that most academic health systems never grasp.

You are aware of the four converging crises in academic medicine: ongoing quality gaps despite medical progress, workforce attrition fueled by organizational issues, financial instability endangering the academic mission, and the seventeen-year delay between evidence development and implementation. You recognize that these challenges are not isolated but are interconnected failures of organizational capacity.

The reason previous transformation efforts failed is not due to a lack of commitment or resources, but because of five common mistakes and overlooking the crucial structural adjustment. These include an obsession with tools without fostering cultural change, siloed excellence without effective knowledge transfer, voluntary participation that allowed opting out, CEO dependency that weakened the process, and attempting culture change through communication instead of structural adjustments. All these issues stem from a deeper underlying problem: the governance void.

You understand the three governance models and how to select the right one. Centralized when consistency is the top priority. Federated when speed and local adaptation are key. Hub-and-spoke is used when both coordination and responsiveness are necessary. It's not about which model is "best," but about which fits your organization and strategic goals best. And you recognize that making a clear choice and executing it completely is more critical than the specific model you pick.

You understand how to approach your first 90 days strategically: ensuring governance is genuine, honestly assessing readiness, developing a vision through dialogue rather than top-down orders, creating quick wins that show value while building capability, establishing a foundation before making announcements, and relying on evidence before generating hype.

You are aware of the three core capabilities that underpin everything else: psychological safety, which allows people to learn from failures without fear; quality improvement mentoring, which develops skills through apprenticeship rather than classroom training; and data-driven learning cycles, which complete the loop from practice, data, insight, to action. Without all three, transformation tends to stall. When all three are in place, the process speeds up.

You are aware of the six pitfalls that can derail transformations even after initial success: declaring victory too soon, tolerating toxic high performers who boost revenue but harm culture, allowing governance to weaken through minor compromises, under-investing in capability renewal, scaling prematurely, and engaging in measurement theater that focuses on metrics instead of results.

Most importantly, learning organizations are not formed by initiatives, consultants, or strategic plans. Instead, they are developed through a systematic process of capability building over a period of 18 to 36 months, with consistent effort. This involves governance structures that grant authority, leadership behaviors that exemplify the desired culture, and infrastructure that supports large-scale learning.

You know what to do. The question is whether you'll actually do it.

THE CHOICE YOU FACE

You cannot go on like this. The crises are not distant threats; they are happening now. Preventable harm persists. Good people are leaving. Margins are shrinking. Evidence grows, but practice remains unchanged. Each month of delay in transformation worsens these issues.

You have three options.

Option one: Continue to act as if everything is fine by launching another improvement initiative with much fanfare. Hire consultants to lead another strategic planning process, announce new priorities at town halls, and form another task force to analyze the issue. Hope that this time, different results will come from the same ineffective approach.

You're familiar with this pattern: eighteen months of effort yielding no real progress. Staff become more cynical as initiatives fail. Metrics temporarily improve but then fall back. Consultants give impressive presentations and then depart. It's just another item on the long list of "things we tried that didn't work."

Option two: Lower your aspirations. Cease claiming to be a learning organization or academic leader. Concentrate solely on financial survival and fundamental operational efficiency. Drop the mission-driven activities that give academic medicine its value but don't produce profit. Turn into a community hospital with a medical school attached.

Some institutions will opt for this route. They will survive financially but will forgo their unique purpose. They may handle payroll but will neglect training future workers, advancing medical research, or supporting safety net populations. It's survival without fulfilling their mission.

Option three: Truly transform. Make the governance decision and carry it out completely. Dedicate eighteen to thirty-six months to developing real learning organization capabilities. Recognize that transformation demands ongoing effort, not quick solutions. Stick to the discipline needed to prevent the common pitfalls that can undermine even well-initiated efforts.

This is the challenging path. You will lose individuals who favor independence over teamwork. Resistance will come from those committed to existing power structures. Expect to make errors and need to adjust your course. You'll allocate resources with no quick payoff. Staying committed through obstacles and doubt will be essential.

However, this is also the sole route that genuinely addresses the crises you're experiencing. It is the only way to achieve long-term enhancements in quality, workforce engagement, financial results, and evidence implementation. Moreover, it is the only approach that allows you to fulfill the promise of academic medicine.

Which path will you choose?

WHAT TRANSFORMATION MAKES POSSIBLE

If you decide to pursue transformation—fully investing in developing your learning organization—here's what could be achievable in the next three to five years.

Your clinical quality metrics will improve steadily and systematically, not just occasionally. This won't happen through isolated pilot projects that lack scalability but through the widespread adoption of evidence-based practices across your entire network. Patients will benefit from consistently higher-quality care, no matter which physician they consult, which unit they are admitted to, or on what day they arrive. Over time, preventable harm will decrease annually as your ability to learn from failures and near-misses enhances.

Your team will become more stable and stronger, with burnout rates decreasing as staff find more meaningful work instead of bureaucratic tasks. Turnover will decrease as top clinicians stay, drawn to an environment that supports their preferred way of practicing medicine. You will draw talented individuals because your reputation as a learning organization makes you a top employer. Early-career faculty will pursue training with you, drawn by a learning environment that offers unique development opportunities.

Your financial performance will be enhanced by systematically eliminating waste and creating value. This approach does not involve random cost cuts that compromise quality, but focuses on identifying the 30-50% of activities that do not contribute to better patient outcomes and removing them. As a result, operating margins will grow, freeing up capacity to invest in mission-critical activities such as education, research, and community benefits that distinguish academic medicine.

Your evidence-to-practice gap will shrink from seventeen years to just months or weeks. Research results from your labs will be implemented in your clinics before competitors are even aware of the evidence. Clinical protocols will be updated immediately as new evidence emerges. Your reputation as an organization that quickly adopts innovation will draw in patients, collaborations, and research funding.

At its core, you'll build organizational resilience to handle any challenges that come your way. This includes adapting to new payment models, competitive threats, regulatory shifts, pandemics, or technologies still unknown. Learning organizations succeed because they can sense environmental changes, test their responses, measure outcomes, and expand what proves effective.

This isn't an idealized dream. It's a documented reality at organizations that have truly developed learning capabilities. Their transformation wasn't quick or straightforward, but it was genuine and enduring.

YOUR FIRST THREE ACTIONS

You've completed this book. You now understand what needs to be done. However, tomorrow morning, you'll still face the same organizational challenges—competing priorities, political dynamics, resource constraints, and resistance to change—as before you started reading.

What do you actually do?

Here are your first three actions.

Action One: Schedule the governance conversation. Within the next two weeks, add an agenda item to your upcoming board or executive team meeting: "Governance model for learning organization development." Come ready with the decision framework from Chapter 3. Lead a clear discussion on organizational priorities, context, and leadership abilities. Ensure you select a governance model—whether centralized, federated, or hub-and-spoke—and document it thoroughly before the meeting ends. Even an imperfect choice is better than delaying; making a decision is crucial.

Action Two: Conduct the honest assessment. Within the next 30 days, conduct a thorough readiness assessment across seven key dimensions: leadership commitment, organizational culture, data infrastructure, QI capacity, communication systems, resources, and external environment. Use the structured framework, but emphasize honesty. Interview opinion leaders willing to speak openly. Focus on actual behaviors rather than aspirational values. Document your findings with detail. Share the results transparently with leadership and the board. If you find you're not yet prepared for transformation, acknowledge it and work on closing the foundational gaps first.

Action Three: Identify your quick wins. Over the next 60 days, choose two to three strategic quick wins that are highly visible, easily measurable, and aligned with your strategy. Focus on manageable problems that can be resolved quickly, avoiding long-term projects that take years to show results. Instead, target opportunities where you can achieve measurable improvements within 90 days. Assign clear leadership, set baseline metrics, and get started. These quick wins will demonstrate that transformation is achievable while generating early momentum.

Three key actions: governance decision, honest assessment, and strategic quick wins. Completing these within 60 days surpasses what most organizations achieve after years of discussing transformation.

Proceed with the 90-day plan outlined in Chapter II:2. Focus on developing the three key capabilities described in Chapter II:3. Be mindful of the mistakes highlighted in Chapter II:4. Stay disciplined, keep investing, and allow enough time for the transformation to evolve from an initiative into a true capability.

THE INVITATION

You don't have to do this alone.

Visit LearningOrgPlaybook.com to access resources supporting your transformation:

- The readiness assessment tools referenced throughout this book
- Vision development worksheets and facilitation guides
- Governance model decision framework
- Implementation checklists for each phase
- Case studies from successful transformations

Most importantly, share your story. Whether you achieve great success, face public struggles, or find approaches we haven't documented, your experience contributes to collective learning. Academic medicine requires more organizations dedicated to real transformation, not just discussing it.

THE FINAL TRUTH

I'll conclude at the starting point—with a truth that may be unsettling but ultimately sets us free.

You understand that your current approach is ineffective. The crises are urgent, and the stakes are significant. Persisting with the same method ensures ongoing failure.

Transformation is challenging but not complex. It depends on transparent governance, honest evaluation, systematic skill development, consistent discipline, and long-term investment. These are well-documented practices validated across many institutions.

The only question is whether you're willing to do what success requires.

Are you prepared to make governance decisions that challenge current power structures? Are you ready to face honest evaluations that uncover uncomfortable truths? Are you willing to invest 18 to 36 months in building capability before declaring success? Are you committed to maintaining discipline even when everything appears to be going well? Are you willing to prioritize the mission over comfort?

If yes, you are all set to start with a clear roadmap, proven practices, and a supportive community. The decision is yours.

If no, be honest about it. Avoid starting initiatives you can't maintain. Don't make promises you won't fulfill. Don't drain your team with unnecessary changes. Recognize that you've settled for the status quo and take responsibility for that choice.

But if you are genuinely prepared to develop real learning organization capabilities, to revolutionize academic medicine for your institution and beyond, and to establish the healthcare system that patients deserve and clinicians wish to work in...

YOUR TRANSFORMATION STARTS NOW.

THE NEXT MOVE IS YOURS.

PART IV

APPENDICES & RESOURCES

READINESS SELF-ASSESSMENT

SEVEN-DIMENSION DIAGNOSTIC TOOL WITH SCORING AND INTERPRETATION GUIDE

Before investing significant resources in learning organization development, assess your organization's current readiness honestly. This self-assessment covers seven critical dimensions. Rate your organization on each item using the scale below, then interpret your results.

Rating Scale:

- 1 = **Strongly Disagree** - This doesn't describe us at all
- 2 = **Disagree** - This describes us minimally
- 3 = **Neutral** - This somewhat describes us
- 4 = **Agree** - This mostly describes us
- 5 = **Strongly Agree** - This fully describes us

Critical instruction: Answer based on actual organizational behavior, not aspirational values or what leadership says. What actually happens, not what should happen.

DIMENSION 1: LEADERSHIP COMMITMENT & CAPABILITY

Rate each statement:

___ Our CEO and executive team personally champion continuous improvement and allocate significant time to transformation efforts, not just delegate to others.

___ Our board understands learning organization principles and actively supports transformation with appropriate resource allocation and governance oversight.

___ Senior leaders model learning behaviors—admitting mistakes, asking for input, changing decisions based on new information.

___ Executive leadership has remained stable (less than one turnover in the past three years in CEO or equivalent positions).

___ Leaders demonstrate systems thinking—understanding how organizational parts interconnect rather than optimizing individual departments.

Dimension 1 Score: ____ / 25

DIMENSION 2: ORGANIZATIONAL CULTURE & CLIMATE

Rate each statement:

___ People feel genuinely safe raising concerns about quality or safety issues without fear of retaliation, even when concerns involve senior physicians or leaders.

___ When mistakes occur, the typical response is curiosity about root causes rather than searching for who to blame.

___ Cross-departmental collaboration happens routinely through standard processes, not requiring heroic individual efforts.

___ Frontline staff regularly contribute ideas for improvement and see those ideas implemented, not ignored.

___ Innovation and experimentation are rewarded even when experiments fail, as long as learning occurs.

Dimension 2 Score: ____ / 25

DIMENSION 3: DATA & TECHNOLOGY INFRASTRUCTURE

Rate each statement:

___ We can extract needed performance data within days, not weeks or months.

___ Our data systems integrate information from multiple sources (EHR, billing, quality databases) into unified views.

___ Frontline teams have direct access to their performance metrics without waiting for central analysts.

___ Our data quality is high enough that people trust metrics and use them for decision-making.

___ We have analytics capability to distinguish meaningful signals from random variation in our metrics.

Dimension 3 Score: ____ / 25

DIMENSION 4: QUALITY IMPROVEMENT CAPACITY

Rate each statement:

___ We have staff trained in quality improvement methodologies (PDSA, Lean, Six Sigma, etc.) who actively use these methods.

___ We have dedicated quality improvement resources (people with protected time, not volunteers doing QI in addition to regular duties).

___ We have completed successful improvement projects that achieved sustained results lasting beyond initial implementation.

___ We have systematic processes for measuring improvement outcomes, not just activity metrics.

___ We have proven ability to spread successful improvements from pilot sites to other areas.

Dimension 4 Score: ____ / 25

DIMENSION 5: COMMUNICATION & KNOWLEDGE SHARING

Rate each statement:

___ Information flows effectively across departmental boundaries through established channels.

___ We have functioning knowledge repositories where innovations and lessons learned are documented and accessible.

___ Regular meetings across the organization have clear purposes, structured agendas, and produce documented decisions.

___ When one unit develops an innovation, other units learn about it through systematic communication, not accidental discovery.

___ Staff report that communication is timely, relevant, and actionable rather than overwhelming or ignored.

Dimension 5 Score: ____ / 25

DIMENSION 6: RESOURCE AVAILABILITY

Rate each statement:

___ We have budget allocated specifically for transformation and improvement work (not expecting transformation to happen with zero incremental investment).

___ Staff have protected time for improvement work built into their roles, not expected to do improvement work on top of full-time clinical or operational duties.

___ We can access external expertise (consultants, coaches, trainers) when needed to supplement internal capability.

___ Our physical and technological infrastructure can support transformation (adequate meeting spaces, collaboration platforms, etc.).

___ Leadership is willing to stop or reduce some current activities to make room for transformation work.

Dimension 6 Score: ____ / 25

DIMENSION 7: EXTERNAL ENVIRONMENT & STAKEHOLDER SUPPORT

Rate each statement:

___ Our community and key external stakeholders (payers, referring physicians, community organizations) support our transformation efforts.

___ Regulatory and accreditation requirements align with rather than conflict with our improvement priorities.

___ Our competitive environment allows time for capability building rather than demanding immediate short-term results.

___ We have partnerships or relationships with other organizations pursuing similar transformation we can learn from.

___ External pressures (financial, regulatory, competitive) create urgency for transformation rather than making it impossible.

Dimension 7 Score: ____ / 25

Seven-Dimension Readiness Assessment

Plot your scores to visualize organizational readiness

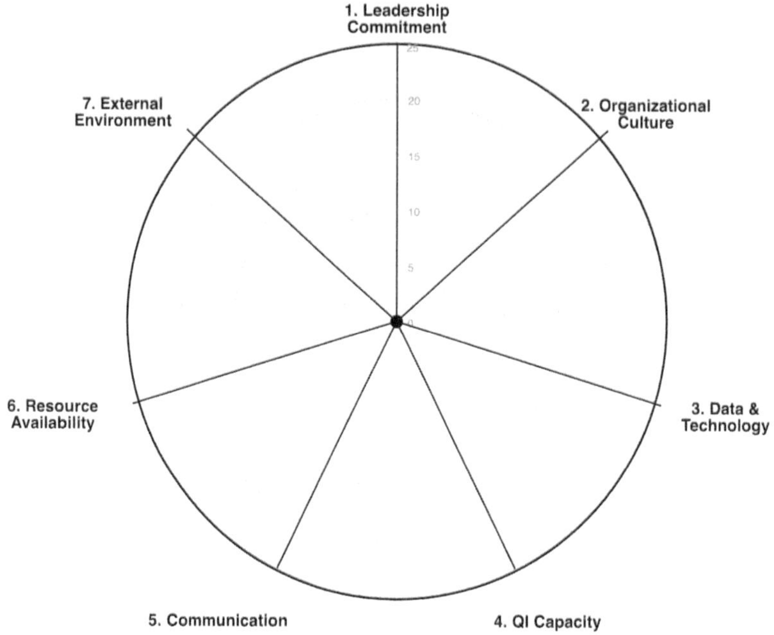

How to Use This Chart

1. Complete the 7-Dimension Readiness Survey (Appendix)
2. Calculate your score for each dimension (out of 25)
3. Plot each score on its corresponding axis:
   - 0 = center point
   - 25 = outer edge
4. Connect the 7 points to create your profile
5. A balanced profile = readiness across all dimensions
6. Spiky profile = specific gaps requiring attention

Interpretation Guide

TOTAL SCORE (sum of all 7):

- 140-175 = HIGH READINESS → Proceed with confidence
- 105-139 = MODERATE → Address gaps while proceeding
- 70-104 = LOW → Build foundation before full transformation
- Below 70 = NOT READY → Focus on stabilization first

ANY dimension scoring below 15 requires immediate attention

SCORING & INTERPRETATION

Calculate your total score: Add all seven dimension scores.

Total Score: ____ / 175

Overall Readiness Assessment:

140-175 (High Readiness): Your organization has a strong foundation for learning organization development. You can proceed with the transformation confident that the basic prerequisites are in place. Focus on: (1) Confirming governance clarity (Chapter II:1), (2) Designing strategic quick wins (Chapter II:2), (3) Building the three essential capabilities systematically (Chapter II:3).

105-139 (Moderate Readiness): Your organization has some foundational elements but significant gaps. You can proceed with the transformation, but you must address the readiness gaps simultaneously. Focus on: (1) Strengthening the weakest dimensions before full-scale transformation, (2) Starting with smaller-scope pilots to build capability, (3) Explicitly planning to develop missing infrastructure as part of the transformation.

70-104 (Low Readiness): Your organization lacks critical prerequisites for successful transformation. Proceeding now will likely fail and create cynicism, making future efforts harder. Instead: (1) Address foundational gaps first—especially leadership commitment and psychological safety, (2) Build basic improvement capacity through targeted skill development, (3) Demonstrate small wins before attempting system-wide transformation, (4) Revisit this assessment in 6-12 months after addressing gaps.

Below 70 (Not Ready): Your organization is not ready for learning organization transformation. Attempting transformation now will fail and damage future change capacity. Honest next steps: (1) Acknowledge current reality without self-deception, (2) Focus on stabilizing basic operations and addressing urgent crises, (3) Build leadership capability and alignment before attempting transformation, (4) Consider external support for developing foundational readiness.

. . .

DIMENSION-SPECIFIC GUIDANCE

If Dimension 1 (Leadership) scored below 15: Transformation cannot succeed without genuine leadership commitment. Before proceeding, secure unambiguous executive and board support. See Chapter II:1, Weeks 1-2 for the governance confirmation process.

If Dimension 2 (Culture) scored below 15: Psychological safety is foundational. Attempting transformation in cultures of blame and fear will fail. Begin culture work before broader transformation. See Chapter II:3, Capability One for psychological safety development.

If Dimension 3 (Data) scored below 15: You cannot learn from practice without data. Invest in data infrastructure before complete transformation. You can still proceed with small pilots while building data capacity, but system-wide transformation requires better infrastructure.

If Dimension 4 (QI Capacity) scored below 15: You lack basic improvement capability. Start with QI training and mentoring for core teams before scaling. See Chapter II:3, Capability Two for mentor network development.

If Dimension 5 (Communication) scored below 15, Knowledge won't spread without a communication infrastructure. Build basic communication channels before attempting system-wide initiatives.

If Dimension 6 (Resources) scored below 15: You cannot transform without investing resources. Either secure necessary resources or scale down ambition to match available investment.

If Dimension 7 (External Environment) scored below 15: External barriers may prevent transformation regardless of internal readiness. Address external constraints or find ways to work within them before embarking on a full-scale transformation.

USING THESE RESULTS

Share honestly with your leadership team and board. Resist the temptation to inflate scores to look better. Honest diagnosis enables effective planning.

Revisit regularly. Assess every six months during active transformation to track progress. Dimensions that scored low initially should show improvement if you're building capability effectively.

Use dimension scores to guide priorities. Focus early transformation efforts on your weakest dimensions since they'll limit overall progress.

Accept the verdict. If your assessment shows you're not ready, accept it. Postponing transformation until you build readiness is better than failing because you proceeded prematurely. Use the assessment to create a readiness development plan, then reassess in 6-12 months.

Remember: This assessment is a diagnostic tool, not a judgment. Low scores don't mean you're bad at healthcare—they indicate you haven't yet built learning organization capability. That's fixable if you're willing to do the work.

RECOMMENDED RESOURCES

HOW TO USE THESE RESOURCES

This list is intentionally selective, not comprehensive. Every resource here offers genuine value for academic health system leaders pursuing learning organization development. I've organized them by type and included brief guidance on when and how to use each.

FOUNDATIONAL BOOKS ON LEARNING ORGANIZATIONS

Peter Senge, *The Fifth Discipline: The Art & Practice of the Learning Organization* (2006)

The original and still essential introduction to learning organization theory. Read this for the five disciplines framework (systems thinking, personal mastery, mental models, shared vision, team learning) that underpins everything else. Dense but worthwhile. Best for: Understanding theoretical foundations.

Peter Senge et al., *The Fifth Discipline Fieldbook* (1994)

Practical companion to *The Fifth Discipline* with tools, exercises, and case studies. More immediately actionable than the original. Read this after the main book when you're ready for implementation guidance. Best for: Translating theory into practice.

Amy Edmondson, *The Fearless Organization: Creating Psychological Safety in the Workplace for Learning, Innovation, and Growth* (2018)

The definitive work on psychological safety—the foundational capability for learning organizations. Essential reading for every leader. Combines research rigor with practical guidance. Best for: Building psychological safety (Chapter 5, Capability One).

David Garvin, Amy Edmondson, Francesca Gino, "Is Yours a Learning Organization?" *Harvard Business Review* (2008)

Excellent diagnostic article with practical assessment framework. Shorter and more accessible than full books. Use this for quick leadership team discussion. Available online. Best for: Executive teams needing condensed overview.

HEALTHCARE-SPECIFIC IMPLEMENTATION

Institute of Medicine, *Best Care at Lower Cost: The Path to Continuously Learning Health Care in America* (2013)

Foundational document for learning health systems concept. Establishes the vision and makes the policy case. Free PDF available online. Best for: Understanding healthcare-specific context and building board support.

Charles P. Friedman, Jeremy C. Wyatt, *Evaluation Methods in Biomedical and Health Informatics* (2006)

Technical but valuable for understanding data infrastructure requirements. Best for:

IT leaders and informatics teams building data-driven learning capability (Chapter 5, Capability Three).

Tom Foley et al., *Learning Health Systems* (2025)

Contemporary synthesis of LHS implementation experiences. Practical case studies from multiple countries. Best for: Understanding real-world implementation challenges and solutions.

Don Berwick, "A User's Manual for the IOM's 'Quality Chasm' Report," *Health Affairs* (2002)

Classic article connecting quality improvement to organizational learning. Older but still relevant. Free online. Best for: Connecting quality improvement to broader transformation.

IMPLEMENTATION SCIENCE AND QUALITY IMPROVEMENT

Gerald Langley et al., *The Improvement Guide: A Practical Approach to Enhancing Organizational Performance* (2009)

The definitive guide to PDSA methodology and improvement science. Technical but essential for QI mentors and leaders. Best for: Building improvement capability (Chapter 5, Capability Two).

Laura J. Damschroder et al., "Fostering Implementation of Health Services Research Findings into Practice: A Consolidated Framework for Advancing Implementation Science," *Implementation Science* (2009)

Academic but valuable framework for understanding implementation barriers. Free online. Best for: Understanding why interventions succeed or fail when scaling.

John P. Kotter, *Leading Change* (1996)

Classic change management framework. Healthcare-agnostic but widely applicable. Quick read with clear eight-step process. Best for: Understanding change leadership fundamentals (especially Chapter 4).

GOVERNANCE AND ORGANIZATIONAL DESIGN

Henry Mintzberg, *Structure in Fives: Designing Effective Organizations* (1993)

Academic but excellent analysis of organizational structures and governance. Helps understand why academic health systems' matrix structures create governance challenges. Best for: Understanding structural options (Chapter 3).

Ram Charan, Dennis Carey, Michael Useem, *Boards That Lead: When to Take Charge, When to Partner, and When to Stay Out of the Way* (2014)

Practical guidance on board governance. Relevant for establishing board role in transformation oversight. Best for: Board members and executives clarifying governance (Chapter 3).

ONLINE RESOURCES AND TOOLS

Institute for Healthcare Improvement (IHI.org)

Extensive free resources including white papers, how-to guides, and recorded webinars on improvement methods. Open School courses provide QI training. Best for: Ongoing education and practical tools.

Agency for Healthcare Research and Quality (AHRQ.gov)
Federal agency providing evidence-based toolkits, quality measures, and implementation guides. All resources free. Best for: Evidence-based practice guidelines and measurement tools.
National Academy of Medicine (NAM.edu)
Policy reports and frameworks including learning health system materials. Free access to major reports. Best for: Understanding policy context and academic perspective.
LearningOrgPlaybook.com (Your Resource Hub)
Companion website to this book providing:

- Downloadable assessment tools and templates
- Implementation checklists for each phase
- Case studies and video interviews
- Monthly implementation calls
- Community forum for peer connection
- Certification programs and consulting services

Best for: Practical implementation support and peer learning.

ACADEMIC JOURNALS (FOR DEEPER DIVES)

Implementation Science (implementationscience.biomedcentral.com)
Open-access journal focused on translating research to practice. Excellent for understanding implementation barriers and enablers.
Learning Health Systems (onlinelibrary.wiley.com/journal/23796146)
Dedicated journal for LHS research and practice. Mix of research and practical guidance.
BMJ Quality & Safety (qualitysafety.bmj.com)
Leading journal for healthcare quality improvement research. Practical and rigorous.
Health Affairs (healthaffairs.org)
Health policy journal with frequent articles on transformation, payment reform, and organizational change. Accessible to non-academics.

PROFESSIONAL ORGANIZATIONS AND NETWORKS

American Association for Physician Leadership (AAPL)
Training and certification for physician leaders. Excellent programs on leading change in healthcare organizations.
American College of Healthcare Executives (ACHE)
Professional organization for healthcare executives with extensive resources on organizational transformation and leadership development.
Healthcare Information and Management Systems Society (HIMSS)
Essential for healthcare IT leaders building data infrastructure for learning organizations.
National Association of Academic Medical Centers (AAMC)

Specific focus on academic health systems with relevant resources on transformation and quality improvement.

WHERE TO START

If you have 1 hour: Read Garvin/Edmondson/Gino HBR article + complete the Readiness Self-Assessment in this book's Appendix.

If you have 1 day: Read Edmondson's *The Fearless Organization* cover to cover. Then revisit Chapter II:3, Capability One.

If you have 1 week: Read Senge's *The Fifth Discipline* + IOM's *Best Care at Lower Cost* + Langley's chapters on PDSA methodology. Then draft your governance model using the Chapter II:1 framework.

If you're building QI capability: Start with Langley's *The Improvement Guide* and IHI Open School courses. Supplement with practical mentoring from experienced improvement leaders.

If you're struggling with specific challenges: Visit LearningOrgPlaybook.com and reach out via email.

FINAL NOTE

Don't let gathering resources turn into procrastination. You already possess what's necessary to begin—this book. Utilize these extra resources to enhance your understanding and support implementation, but avoid delaying action while seeking more content.

Effective learning stems from active practice, reflection, and adjustments. Begin applying what you learn. Use these resources to address specific challenges or to gain more in-depth knowledge in particular areas.

Your transformation begins with action, not more reading.

ABOUT THE AUTHOR

Nabil Zary, MD, PhD, is a physician, educator, and organizational transformation advisor who has spent over two decades helping academic health systems build the capacity to learn faster than they fail.

His career began at the intersection of medicine and technology as Technical Director of the Wallenberg Global Learning Network at Stanford University. He went on to direct the Centre for Learning and Knowledge at Karolinska Institutet in Sweden, where he led educational innovations deployed across 38 universities. In Singapore, he founded the Games for Health Innovations Centre at Nanyang Technological University's Lee Kong Chian School of Medicine. Today, he advises health systems internationally on learning organization development.

Through leadership roles spanning Sweden, the United States, and Singapore, and consulting engagements across Europe, the Middle East, and Latin America, Dr. Zary has observed a consistent pattern: academic health systems invest heavily in transformation, yet most initiatives fail. Not for lack of resources, but because organizations misunderstand what it means to become a *learning* organization. They purchase technology without changing culture. They train individuals without building systems. They announce strategies without rethinking governance.

This book distills those insights into an actionable framework for leaders ready to do transformation differently.

Dr. Zary holds an MD and PhD from Karolinska Institutet and has contributed to governance and standards development for the Association of American Medical Colleges (AAMC). His research on learning innovation has been published extensively in peer-reviewed journals and cited in World Health Organization initiatives.

linkedin.com/in/nabilzary
facebook.com/nabilzary
x.com/nabilzary
youtube.com/@nabilzary
tiktok.com/@nabilzary
pinterest.com/nabilzaryauthor
instagram.com/nabilzary
amazon.com/author/nabilzary

www.ingramcontent.com/pod-product-compliance
Lightning Source LLC
Chambersburg PA
CBHW051400240926
51852CB00002B/70
* 9 7 8 9 6 9 9 8 9 3 5 4 4 *